Play Therapy Theories and Perspectives

This book explores the multitude of thoughts, theories, opinions, methods, and approaches to play therapy in order to highlight the unity and diversity of theory and perspective in the field.

Each chapter is a common question related to play therapy to which ten established and experienced play therapists share their thoughts, theoretical perspectives, and opinions. The key characteristics of a well-trained play therapist, the role of technology in play therapy, the importance of speaking the client's language, and many more frequently asked play therapy questions and topics are explored. The reader will learn about the umbrella of play therapy thought and practice and connect with perspectives that might align with their own theoretical preferences.

This book will be of interest to a wide range of mental health professionals working with children and adolescents. Those new to play therapy and those who are seasoned veterans will appreciate, value, and hopefully be challenged by the differing viewpoints surrounding many play therapy topics.

Robert Jason Grant, EdD, LPC, RPT-S, ACAS, owns and operates the Aut-Play Therapy Clinic in Southwest Missouri. He is the creator of AutPlay® Therapy and a multi-published author of several articles, chapters, and books. He is an international presenter and keynote speaker and currently serves as a board member for the Association for Play Therapy.

Jessica Stone, PhD, RPT-S, is a licensed psychologist working in a private practice setting in Colorado. She has been a practitioner, professor, presenter, mentor, and author for more than 25 years. She is the co-creator of the Virtual Sandtray App for iPad (VSA) and the Virtual Sandtray for Virtual Reality (VSA-VR). Dr. Stone has numerous publications to date including Integrating Technology into Modern Therapies, Game Play, and Digital Play Therapy.

Clair Mellenthin, LCSW, RPT-S, is an international speaker, author, and Registered Play Therapist Supervisor. She holds a Master's Degree in Social Work from the University of Southern California. She is currently the Director of Child & Adolescents at Wasatch Family Therapy and an adjunct faculty member at the University of Southern California MSW program.

Play Therapy Theories and Perspectives

A Collection of Thoughts in the Field

Edited by Robert Jason Grant,
Jessica Stone, and Clair Mellenthin

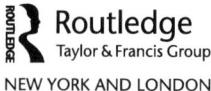

Routledge
Taylor & Francis Group

NEW YORK AND LONDON

First published 2021
by Routledge
52 Vanderbilt Avenue, New York, NY 10017

and by Routledge
2 Park Square, Milton Park, Abingdon, Oxon, OX14 4RN

Routledge is an imprint of the Taylor & Francis Group, an informa business

© 2021 Taylor & Francis

The right of Robert Jason Grant, Jessica Stone, and Clair Mellenthin
to be identified as the authors of the editorial material, and of the
authors for their individual chapters, has been asserted in accordance
with sections 77 and 78 of the Copyright, Designs and Patents
Act 1988.

Library of Congress Cataloging-in-Publication Data
Names: Grant, Robert Jason, 1971– editor. |
Stone, Jessica (Child psychologist) editor. | Mellenthin, Clair, editor.
Title: Play therapy theories and perspectives: diversity of thought in the field /
edited by Robert Jason Grant, Jessica Stone, Clair Mellenthin.
Identifiers: LCCN 2020016330 (print) | LCCN 2020016331 (ebook) |
ISBN 9780367418380 (hardback) | ISBN 9780367418373 (paperback) |
ISBN 9780367816452 (ebook)
Subjects: LCSH: Play therapy.
Classification: LCC RJ505.P6 P5468 2021 (print) |
LCC RJ505.P6 (ebook) | DDC 618.92/891653—dc23
LC record available at https://lccn.loc.gov/2020016330
LC ebook record available at https://lccn.loc.gov/2020016331

ISBN: 978-0-367-41838-0 (hbk)
ISBN: 978-0-367-41837-3 (pbk)
ISBN: 978-0-367-81645-2 (ebk)

Typeset in Goudy
by codeMantra

Contents

    Respect to Client Ages?   198

    Conclusion   207
    CLAIR MELLENTHIN AND JESSICA STONE

    Index   209

Contributors

Dr. Jeff Ashby, RPT-S, is a professor in the Department of Counseling and Psychological Services at Georgia State University. He is a licensed psychologist, a diplomate of the American Board of Professional Psychology, and a Registered Play Therapist-Supervisor. He is the codirector of Georgia State's Center for the Study of Stress, Trauma, and Resilience and the former director of Play Therapy Training Institute.

Robert Jason Grant, EdD, LPC, RPT-S, ACAS, owns and operates the AutPlay Therapy Clinic in Southwest Missouri. He is the creator of AutPlay® Therapy and he is a multipublished author of several articles, book chapters, and books including the following best-selling books: *AutPlay® Therapy for Children and Adolescents on the Autism Spectrum, Play-Based Interventions for Autism Spectrum Disorder, Understanding Sensory Processing Challenges, A Workbook for Children and Teens*, and *Understanding Autism Spectrum Disorder, A Workbook for Children and Teens*. Dr. Grant is the recipient of the Association for Play Therapy's Service award and Missouri Association for Play Therapy's Outstanding Play Therapist award. He is an international presenter and keynote speaker, and currently serves as a board member for the Association for Play Therapy.

Heidi Gerard Kaduson, PhD, RPT-S, specializes in evaluation and intervention services for children with a variety of behavioral, emotional, and learning problems. She is past president of the Association for Play Therapy and director of The Play Therapy Training Institute, Inc., in Monroe Township, New Jersey. She has lectured internationally on play therapy, attention-deficit/hyperactivity disorder, and learning disabilities. Dr. Kaduson has authored chapters and coedited books, including *Game Play Interventions for Children with Attention-deficit Hyperactivity Disorder, Release Play Therapy, Play Therapy Across the Lifespan, Play Therapy for Children with Attention-deficit Hyperactivity Disorder, The Playing Cure, Short-Term Play Therapy, 3rd Edition, 101 Favorite Play Therapy Techniques, 101 More Favorite Play Therapy Techniques, 101 Favorite Play Therapy Techniques, Volume III*, and *Contemporary Play Therapy*. She maintains a private practice in child psychotherapy in Monroe Township, New Jersey.

Jennifer Lefebre, PsyD, RPT-S, TCTSY-F, is a clinical psychologist, Registered Play Therapist-Supervisor, and trauma-sensitive yoga facilitator. She is the president-elect for the New England Association for Play Therapy. Her clinical and research interests focus on the assessment and treatment of children, adolescents, adults, and families whose lives have been impacted by complex trauma. Dr. Lefebre has extensive experience working with young children (0–5), adult survivors of severe childhood abuse and neglect, first responders, and combat veterans. Dr. Lefebre is the clinical director at Healing the Child Within, a holistic trauma center in northwestern Connecticut which integrates psychotherapy, yoga, play, and expressive arts therapies into the treatment of complex trauma. She also provides clinical supervision and play therapy consultation throughout New England and online, and an adjunct faculty member at several universities, teaching both at the undergraduate and graduate level. In addition to being an experienced play therapist and professor, Dr. Lefebre is a sought-after expert for speaking engagements, podcasts, and webinars on the topics of play therapy and complex childhood trauma.

Clair Mellenthin, LCSW, RPT-S, is an international speaker, author, and Registered Play Therapist-Supervisor. She holds a master's degree in Social Work from the University of Southern California. Throughout her career, she has specialized in providing play therapy to children, teens, and their families. She is currently the director of Child & Adolescents at Wasatch Family Therapy. Ms. Mellenthin frequently presents professional play therapy and family therapy professional trainings on Attachment-Centered Play Therapy, Family, and Trauma issues, both nationally and internationally. Ms. Mellenthin is a sought-after supervisor, training graduate students and interns in play therapy, and an adjunct faculty member at the University of Southern California MSW program. She is the past president of the Utah Association for Play Therapy and remains an active member on the board of directors. She is the author of *Attachment Centered Play Therapy*; *Play Therapy: Engaging & Powerful Techniques for the Treatment of Childhood Disorders*; and *My Many Colors of Me Workbook*, and has authored several chapters and articles. In addition to being an experienced play therapist and professor, Ms. Mellenthin frequently presents professional play therapy and family therapy trainings, and appears on local and national TV and radio as an expert on children and family issues.

Akiko J. Ohnogi, PsyD, utilizes play therapy with all of her clients, including very young children, adolescents, and adults, and specializes in treatment of children, trauma survivors, and multicultural families. She is cofounder of Japan Association for Play Therapy, which provides play therapy training to mental health practitioners, and post-trauma support for survivors, throughout Japan. Dr. Ohnogi has several publications in the United States and Japan, and has provided workshops in the United States,

Ireland, England, Argentina, and Japan. She taught play therapy to graduate students at her undergraduate alma mater and was school counselor of her middle school alma mater. She has been in private practice in Tokyo since 2000.

Mary Anne Peabody, EdD, LCSW, RPT-S, is currently an associate professor at the University of Southern Maine, a licensed clinical social worker, Registered Play Therapist-Supervisor, and past K-12 school counselor. She served as chair of the National Association for Play Therapy, president of the Maine branch of Play Therapy and recently was the recipient of the Distinguished Service Award from the Association for Play Therapy. She currently serves on the *International Journal of Play Therapy* editorial board, the Foundation Board of Play Therapy, and the New England Play therapy branch board. She presents internationally and has published extensively in the field of play therapy, play, and leadership.

Dee Ray, PhD, LPC-S, NCC, RPT-S, is distinguished teaching professor and Elaine Millikan Mathes Professor in Early Childhood Education in the Counseling Program and director of the Center for Play Therapy at the University of North Texas. Dr. Ray has published over 100 articles, chapters, and books in the field of play therapy, specializing in research specifically examining the process and effects of Child Centered Play Therapy. Dr. Ray is author of *A Therapist's Guide to Development: The Extraordinarily Normal Years*, *Advanced Play Therapy: Essential Conditions, Knowledge, and Skills for Child Practice*, and *Child Centered Play Therapy Treatment Manual*, and coauthor of *Group Play Therapy* and *Child Centered Play Therapy Research*. She is founding editor of the *Journal of Child and Adolescent Counseling* and an American Counseling Association Fellow, and is a recipient of the American Counseling Association Don Dinkmeyer Social Interest Award, Association for Humanistic Counseling Educator Award, Association for Play Therapy Outstanding Research Award, Top 25 Women Professors in Texas Award, and many others.

Jessica Stone, PhD, RPT-S, is a licensed psychologist working in a private practice setting in Colorado. She has been a practitioner, professor, presenter, mentor, and author for more than 25 years. Dr. Stone's interest in therapeutic digital tools, specifically using virtual reality, tablets, and consoles, has culminated in clinical mental health use and research for mental health, medical, and crisis settings. She is the cocreator of the Virtual Sandtray App for iPad (VSA) and the Virtual Sandtray for Virtual Reality (VSA-VR). Dr. Stone has numerous publications to date including *Integrating Technology into Modern Therapies*, *Game Play*, and *Digital Play Therapy*, and numerous chapters in a variety of books. She has served as the president of the California Association for Play Therapy branch and the Leadership Academy chair (the Association for Play Therapy Nominations Committee), and is a member of the AutPlay Advisory Board.

Daniel Sweeney, PhD, RPT-S, is the founder and director of the Northwest Center for Play Therapy Studies. He is also a tenured professor of counseling and clinical director of the Marriage, Couple and Family Counseling program in the Graduate School of Counseling at George Fox University. Dr. Sweeney is a former member of the board of directors and past president of the Association for Play Therapy, a Registered Play Therapist-Supervisor (RPT-S), and maintains a small private practice. Daniel has extensive experience in working with children, couples, and families in a variety of settings, including therapeutic foster care, community mental health, private practice, and pastoral counseling. He has presented at regional, national, and international conferences on the topics of play therapy, sand tray therapy, filial therapy, couple and family therapy, and trauma interventions.

Foreword

This foreword has the dubious distinction of being written during the 2020 COVID-19 global pandemic which has challenged and distressed us all. The situation we face together is unpredictable and shocking, and the number of individuals infected, sick, recovering, or dying from this virus has been steadily increasing. The scientists tell us the virus will lose its power over time, and yet the devastation will most certainly be far-reaching. As many have articulated, the impact of this virus will persist in unimaginable ways for years to come. And yet in the midst of all this, the human spirit soars.

It's hard to find relief and reassurance amidst this intense human crisis. And yet I have seen many things that are uplifting. As Fred Rogers once said, "When I was a boy and I would see scary things in the news, my mother would say to me, 'Look for the helpers. You will always find people who are helping.'" Nowhere has this been more evident than in the play therapy community. It's therefore compelling to write this foreword in the context of our current experiences.

Origins of play therapy can be traced back to the early 1900s. Play therapy as a field became more formalized and established by forward-thinking clinicians in 1982 with Charles Schaefer and Kevin O'Conner founding the Association for Play Therapy and Garry Landreth, Louise Guerney, and others envisioning a movement of individuals joined by a common interest in play as a therapeutic model. In 1983, a small group of people gathered to have the first national play therapy conference in New York. I believe the earliest gathering included around 50 professionals, and the National Association for Play Therapy Conference has now grown to approximately 1,200 attendees annually. Initially the association started with 50 members and currently has over 7,500 members. The National Association for Play Therapy Conference is an event that highlights the past, present, and future visions for our growing professional field, and the Association has developed standards of practice, ethical standards, and a rigorous credentialing process for professionals proving play therapy's efficiency and/or pursuing a play therapy credential.

During this time of crisis, I remind people that the Chinese characters that depict the word "crisis" are "danger and opportunity." The play therapy community is acknowledging the danger and creating ample opportunities as well. Those opportunities will occur during tele-health with children and families, as therapists and clients rediscover each other in different ways, and find meaningful ways to connect. I am watching my colleagues, new and seasoned, rise to the occasion buoyed by their hearts and generous spirits. It's a time to celebrate our play therapy community and the many voices that have risen. As always, the voices are diverse, varied, and multifaceted. There are as many suggestions as there are theories, and the guidance is overwhelming.

The fact that many voices have risen to speak from different vantage points, and to suggest flexible, alternative approaches for meeting the needs of children and families, is nothing new. The play therapy field has always been exciting in its evolution. The Association for Play Therapy recently developed and published a list of the seminal theories of play therapy that are valid and reliable methods for guiding the practice of play therapy. Those foundational theories include psychoanalytic, behavioral, humanistic, Adlerian, developmental, and Jungian, to name a few. These theories are well articulated and established, and ongoing research and practice efforts are underfoot to target key issues that might benefit from different forms of play therapy, such as ADHD, OCD, anxiety and depression, anger and dysregulation, gender identity concerns, suicidality, and other symptomatic behaviors or conditions. In addition, play therapists have documented methods for providing services to specific target groups: traumatized children, witnesses of interpersonal violence, children with sexual behavior problems, children on the spectrum, children with anxious attachment behaviors, developmental delays, and so on. And still other play therapists have developed and shared expertise on working with infants and toddlers, elementary-aged, or teen clients, as well as couples and families. And thus, the plethora of approaches and interventions continue, likely falling into one of the seminal theories, and allowing therapists to customize their techniques to meet the unique needs of the target groups mentioned, and those that will emerge.

For the most part, play therapists demonstrate the ability to "play well with others," often utilizing a multimodal approach that is integrative. Others, however, prefer a purist approach and stay on the lane that is paved by one primary theory. Charles Schaefer and Athena Drewes wrote about 20 change agents of play that inherently create positive therapeutic outcome, and these change agents are in the forefront of how many play therapists approach the provision of services. As play therapists seek to explain and understand the variables that heighten the potential for play therapy to help children and their families, play therapy research has provided another foundational layer for the work we do, increasing our credibility in the professional community. I know the play therapy community is indebted to the pioneering research efforts of Sue Bratton and Dee Ray, to name just a couple. Others are working diligently to continue in the tradition of science informing practice and vice versa.

As we think through the current complexion of contemporary play therapy, the excitement among play therapists to keep suggesting innovative ideas, and the desire to share positive treatment outcomes with others, some considerations must be acknowledged. It is critical to take the time to try out recommendations, build a foundation of experience and/or scientific study, and ensure that ideas are tested and retested. In addition, it's important for play therapists to assert approach similarities, as well as the nuanced differences. In this regard, this book could not arrive at a better time.

When Dr. Grant contacted me about his book idea, with an invitation to provide a foreword, I was delighted to participate. He described an ingenious approach of posing commonly asked questions and inviting ten seasoned play therapists to respond. The ten play therapy authors represented multiple theories and seemed uniquely suited to convey their points of view. This book project sounded like a labor of love and an open letter to the play therapy community.

After reading the book, I'm filled with inspiration and joy! It was so much fun to read responses to some basic and deep questions, and recognize not only the common factors that are shared but the ways in which the authors revealed a bird's eye view of how their behavior is shaped by thoughtful consideration. Each author carefully deliberated each question providing the readers with nuance and depth, which included the intersection between personal and professional experience. I honestly feel like I know the authors a little bit better by reading their responses throughout the book. Reading it provoked introspection, laughter, and feelings of warmth and camaraderie. It reminded me of many situations I encountered when I was working directly with children and families, and many of the situations that therapists bring to consultation and/or supervision. Most importantly, the book demonstrates what we are all finding critical at this moment: We need to support each other's differing approaches and recognize the ways in which they are solidly grounded in theory. Without that basic construct, we will flutter wildly, without intention and without focus. Our profession is as strong as each of its participants and whether we want to be or not, we are all ambassadors of play therapy. This book offers varied powerful suggestions for practicing play therapy in an ethical, goal-oriented, and purposeful manner. The topics are varied as you will see in the Table of Contents and include a wide range of dialogues about ethics, supervision, boundaries, intersectionality, technology, confidentiality, practicing in urban and rural settings, social media, theory and application, and other fascinating issues. The questions chosen for discussion are ones that currently pop up in most workshops and conferences.

There are equal servings of serious and light communications in the book, as well as occasional calls to action. There are intimate communications about each author and what has led them to their convictions. There are little surprises (Who knew, for example, that Daniel Sweeney does not describe himself as a child-centered play therapist?) and contextual information about diverse practice settings and communities.

I am grateful to Robert for having the vision for this book. I am also grateful for Jessica and Clair's contributions, for their collective crafting of this publication and inviting interesting and informative authors, and for being a part of the new generation of thoughtful and innovative play therapists.

– Eliana Gil, PhD, RPT-S, ATR

Acknowledgments

Thank you to my family who provide support and encouragement in all my writing endeavors and allow me to write in my "extra" time. I could not have written this book without their patience and understanding. Thank-you to all the contributors – your thoughtfulness in responding to these play therapy questions is truly the highlight of this book. Thank-you to Stars for Autism for the inspiration and thank-you to all the play therapists who have encouraged me along the way – I love our field of play therapy!

– Robert Jason Grant

I really appreciate the opportunity that Dr. Grant offered to me when he approached me with this fantastic project. Editing with Dr. Grant and Ms. Mellenthin has been a wonderful experience. The contributors have provided us with amazing responses and have made this text a resource for veteran and new play therapists alike. My family has sacrificed time and some decent meals to allow me to contribute to this project and I cannot thank them enough.

– Jessica Stone

I am so grateful to Matt and our kids for always being supportive of my professional endeavors and being willing to share our time together to allow for this book to be written. Thank-you to our editor Amanda Devine for your support in our ideas to bring a whole new kind of book to the play therapy field. I am so grateful to my many friends and mentors in our field whose voices helped me to find mine. A special thanks to the contributors to this book who were willing to be vulnerable and share their personal experiences, thoughts, and perspectives. I love our work and am so grateful for the many dedicated play therapists who are working to make the world a better place!

– Clair Mellenthin

Introduction

Robert Jason Grant

The Association for Play Therapy (2020) defines play therapy as "the systematic use of a theoretical model to establish an interpersonal process wherein trained play therapists use the therapeutic powers of play to help clients prevent or resolve psychosocial difficulties and achieve optimal growth and development." Play therapy embodies an umbrella term as play therapy can refer to a large number of treatment methods, all applying the therapeutic benefits of play. Many theories, approaches, and methods of play therapy exist, and much has been identified, researched, written about, and proposed as play therapy.

Currently, the Association for Play Therapy recognizes ten seminal and/ or historically significant play therapy theories and approaches. The list includes Adlerian, child-centered, cognitive-behavioral, developmental (Viola Brody), ecosystemic, filial, Gestalt, Jungian, object-relations, and Theraplay®. Beyond these ten recognized, there exists several established and emerging play therapy theories, approaches, and modalities such as sand tray therapy, family play therapy, experiential play therapy, expressive play therapy, relationship play therapy, first play, AutPlay therapy, digital play therapy, TraumaPlay, synergetic play therapy, and animal-assisted play therapy – to name a few. Many play therapists self-identify as an integrative play therapist (combining different therapeutic methods, interventions, and approaches to best fit the needs of the individual client) or prescriptive play therapist (selecting and implementing a particular play therapy approach that research has indicated is likely to be the most effective for a specific problem or symptom). The possibilities of what "play therapy" might mean or look like in implementation are so varied that I often teach parents if someone tells you they do play therapy, the next question you should ask is, "What type of play therapy do you do?"

One unifying feature throughout the myriad of play therapy approaches is Schaefer and Drewes' (2014) 20 core change agents of the therapeutic powers of play. These powers refer to the specific change agents in which play initiates, facilitates, or strengthens the therapeutic effect. Play powers act as mediators that positively influence the desired change in the client (Barron & Kenny, 1986) and provide the foundational framework for the clinical understanding and use of play therapy (VanFleet & Faa-Thompson, 2017). The 20 core change agents include self-expression, access to the unconscious, direct teaching, indirect teaching, catharsis, abreaction, positive emotions, counterconditioning fears, stress inoculation, stress management, therapeutic relationship, attachment, social competence, empathy, creative problem-solving, resiliency, moral development, accelerated psychological development, self-regulation, and self-esteem. Under the umbrella of play therapy, the therapeutic powers of play can be recognized throughout various theories and approaches. Some powers may be more evident or primary in some theories versus others, but certainly the therapeutic powers of play serve as a unifying component in the vast world of play therapy. This book does not capture all the play therapy theories, approaches, and methods that currently exist, but it does provide a snapshot of the variety that permeates across perspectives.

Each contributor to this book has amassed several years working in the field of play therapy. Nine professionals are from the United States and have obtained the credential of Registered Play Therapist-Supervisor (RPT-S), one professional is an international play therapist and cofounder of the Japan Association for Play Therapy – all ten have all trained, presented, and written about play therapy. They each have their unique voice which serves to accomplish one of the original goals of the book – to provide a small snapshot into understanding diversity of thought in the play therapy community. Additionally, there was a desire to buttress the diversity with the unity that manifests across play therapy perspectives. Those who venture into the world of play therapy quickly realize that there is more than one thought, theory, opinion, approach, and method to "doing" play therapy, but the power lies in the appreciation of the integration of diversity and unity which serves to deepen play therapy application.

Across contributors' different theoretical orientations, experiences, and beliefs about play and play therapy, there exists a unity of thought about many aspects that binds the play therapy community. Among the unifying beliefs included are the power of therapeutic relationship, the emphasis on quality supervision, the need for continuous training and growth, the importance of play and speaking the child's language, and the passion about protecting the integrity of the play therapy field. It could be argued that the unifying features in play therapy are the most fundamental and most important when serving children and families. What brings play therapists together are typically the most thoughtful and effective components of therapy.

Although unity in play therapy is evident, there still exists diversity in approach and thought. Diversity and differences do not have to be considered problematic. In fact, they are assets that enrich the professional experience. Diversity and differing perspectives contribute to the strengths in creating the best possible format in which to provide therapy. For the play therapist to fully benefit from the variance of perspectives, the following should be considered:

1 There should be a commitment to respecting differences.
2 There should be an understanding and appreciation for shared values and what unifies us as a play therapy community.
3 There should be an understanding that diversity of play therapy implementation parallels the diversity needs of clients, ultimately validating play therapy as a treatment modality for all children.
4 There should be a commitment to encouraging diversity in perspective as opposed to devaluing and limiting perspectives.
5 There should be marked celebration of the connectedness in play therapy regardless of theoretical differences.

The value of perspective is one of the principles that inspired me to create this book. Several years ago, I was asked to join the board of a nonprofit organization called Stars for Autism. The creators of this organization consisted of a group of autism authors who had written a book together called *Stars in Her Eyes: Navigating the Maze of Childhood Autism*. I remember reading this book and not only gaining valuable knowledge about autism but being intrigued with the format. There were five authors, each from a different professional and personal background but all related to autism. One of the authors was a speech therapist, another a special education director, another a teacher, another a parent, and another a community advocate. The book contained several popular topics/questions about autism (each chapter of the book was a different topic/question) and each of the authors responded to the topic/question from their own experiences, perspective, and opinions. I found this format not only interesting but valuable as I was able to glean multiple perspectives about some of the most common questions related to autism. Before I had finished this book, I was processing how valuable this format would be in a play therapy book. I begin to envision a book reference where several established play therapists shared their perspective on a variety of common play therapy topics and questions.

My journey in learning and appreciation for the variety of theories and approaches in play therapy guided the formation of this book. Each chapter is a common question related to play therapy, and all ten contributors share their thoughts, theoretical perspectives, and opinions on each question. Those new to play therapy and those who are seasoned veterans will appreciate, value, and possibly be challenged by the differing viewpoints surrounding many play therapy topics. This book builds on the work of viewing differing perspectives as an asset while celebrating the unifying features that connect those in the field of play therapy.

References

Association for Play Therapy (2020). *Play therapy makes a difference.* https://www.a4pt. org/page/PTMakesADifference.

Barron, R., & Kenny, D. (1986). The moderator-mediator variable distinction in social psychological research: Conceptual, strategic, and statistical considerations. *Journal of Personality and Social Psychology, 5,* 1173–1182.

Schaefer, C. E., & Drewes, A. A. (2014). *The therapeutic powers of play: 20 core agents of change.* Wiley and Sons.

VanFleet, R., & Faa-Thompson, T. (2017). *Animal assisted play therapy.* Professional Resource Press.

Part I

Perspective

1 Do You Have a Primary Play Therapy Theory or Approach You Use the Most and Why?

Jeff Ashby, PhD, RPT-S

I self-identify as an Adlerian play therapist (Kottman & Meany-Walen, 2016) and naturally resonate with the teleological, strengths-based approach of Adlerian play therapy (AdPT). I began my career treating primarily adults and adolescents and only came to play therapy mid-career. In this transition I was mentored by Dr. Terry Kottman, PhD, the originator of Adlerian play therapy (e.g., Kottman, 1999). While Kottman is the original author and developer of AdPT, as a supervisor and consultant, she was (and is) gracious in helping play therapists understand and develop their own style. She encourages folks to practice from the theoretical perspective that complements their style and allows them to conceptualize client issues from a coherent and consistent framework. In describing my natural assumptions and beliefs about human beings, and how I conceptualized and formulated treatment plans for adult and adolescent clients, Dr. Kottman would consistently point out, "That's Adlerian".

In addition to a comfort in conceptualizing from an Adlerian perspective, the structure of AdPT, including the four identified phases of therapy, combined with the flexibility of approach (e.g., a combination of directive and nondirective techniques), has allowed me the freedom to develop my own style while remaining theoretically consistent. AdPT rests on several tenets of Adlerian psychology. These are as follows: (1) people are self-determining and creative, (2) people perceive reality subjectively, (3) behavior is purposeful and goal-directed, (4) people have a need to belong and are best understood in the context of their social settings (e.g., family), and (5) because of the common separation between self-perception and one's ideal self, people have a tendency toward feeling inferior (Ansbacher & Ansbacher, 1956; Kottman & Meany-Walen, 2016). These assumptions, in combination with other Adlerian principles, offer me a framework to understand the child, frame the child's distress, and formulate a plan to intervene. They help me decide what to do next and give me a roadmap when I'm lost with a client.

My goal in play therapy is to understand clients in terms of their lifestyle (Kottman & Meany-Walen, 2016). Lifestyle is an Adlerian construct that includes a person's beliefs about self, others, the world, and behaviors based on those beliefs (Carlson et al., 2005). The process of AdPT includes four phases: (a) an initial phase of building the relationship, (b) a phase devoted to an exploration and understanding the client's lifestyle, (c) a third phase designed to help the client develop insight into their lifestyle, and (d) a final phase in which the play therapist facilitates client reorientation/reeducation (Kottman & Meany-Walen, 2016). In AdPT, I can utilize a wide range of techniques, depending on the phase of treatment, presenting problem, and lifestyle assessment of the client, and include other members of the client's system.

Robert Jason Grant EdD, RPT-S

I primarily use AutPlay therapy. It is an integrative family play therapy approach that is focused on working with children and adolescents with autism spectrum disorder and related conditions. Theoretical foundations of AutPlay include behavioral therapy methodology and play therapy theories such as filial play therapy, Theraplay, cognitive behavioral play therapy, and child-centered play therapy (Grant, 2017). Most of the population that I work with in a private practice setting are children and adolescents diagnosed with autism or a related condition. I use AutPlay therapy because it is designed for the unique needs and issues that children with autism present.

I began my play therapy journey learning about child-centered play therapy (Landreth, 1991). I have found that most play therapists seem to begin with this theory and consider it a foundational approach. Child-centered play therapy was the first play therapy theory that I learned fully and felt the most competent implementing. I then began to learn other theories and approaches. Throughout the years, I have systematically become an integrative play therapist. I often integrate various play therapy theories and approaches, along with protocols outside of play therapy theories such as social stories, autism movement therapy, and EMDR.

Integrative therapy combines different therapeutic tools and approaches to fit the needs of the individual client. Integrative play therapy is based in integrative therapy theory and philosophy. The play therapist explores methods for blending the best play therapy theories and treatment techniques to resolve the most common psychological disorders of childhood (Drewes, Bratton, & Schaefer, 2011). An example would be that I might be implementing AutPlay therapy protocol and decide that a client would benefit from and respond well to a social story; thus, I would integrate a social story into the AutPlay protocol. This would require that I am knowledgeable in AutPlay therapy, social stories, and the process of integrating protocols.

I would encourage those beginning play therapy to start with learning foundational approaches such as child-centered play therapy (Landreth, 1991) and filial therapy (VanFleet, 2014). Once the therapist feels comfortable with those approaches, I would encourage them to explore other play therapy theories and approaches moving into learning about integrative and prescriptive approaches, ultimately finding their fit in terms of what approach(es) they feel the most comfortable with and what seems to best fit the clients they are serving.

A caution about integrative and prescriptive approaches – the therapist should be well trained and knowledgeable in the theories they are prescribing or integrating. The therapist should not try to be prescriptive or integrative with theories or approaches in which they are not fully knowledgeable.

Heidi Gerard Kaduson, PhD, RPT-S

When I started my career (almost 30 years ago) I was taught like most play therapists that play therapy was done using the nondirective method. I became increasingly aware, however, of how it did not fit many of the children I was treating who were referred for behavior difficulties. I had been trained in all of the theories and began to use a more prescriptive approach in order to meet the needs of each individual child. The prescriptive approach was first introduced to play therapists in the book *The Playing Cure: Individualized Play Therapy for Specific Childhood Disorders* (Kaduson, Cangelosi, & Schaefer, 1997). This approach uses the application of the therapeutic powers of play (Schaefer & Drewes, 2014) to the common psychological disorders of children and adolescents.

Prescriptive play therapy is founded on a set of basic principles that serve as fundamental cornerstones of the approach (Kaduson, Cangelosi, & Schaefer, 2020): differential therapeutics (some interventions are more effective than others for certain disorders); eclecticism (employing elements from a range of theories and/or techniques with the aim of establishing an intervention tailored to a particular client's characteristics and situation); integrative psychotherapy (blending together the healing elements from different schools of play therapy into one combined approach for the treatment of a specific client); and prescriptive matching (matching the most effective play interventions to each specific disorder or presenting problem (Norcross, 1991). However, it also includes having the clinician select a therapeutic change agent that is designed to reduce or eliminate the cause of the problem, as well as an Individualized Treatment (tailoring the intervention to meet the needs of a specific client – not to just treat the presenting problem but the person who is suffering from it). Empirically supported play therapy treatments are listed in Table 1.1 (Kaduson et al., 1997, 2020).

Whenever a preschooler is referred for treatment, I will start with a nondirective, or child-centered approach. However, if the child needs more assistance in order to use pretend play to heal himself, or is past the preoperational stage of development where pretend play is natural, then I will decide what type of interventions are needed and which theoretical approach can best assist the child to play and work through psychological difficulties. I truly believe that every child has the ability to heal through play. My approach stems from a number of play therapy theories and techniques which informs the selection of an intervention best suited to overcome the client's presenting problems. I tailor this therapeutic intervention to the characteristics and preferences of the individual client to achieve an individualized approach.

Table 1.1 Interventions with Empirical Support for Specific Childhood Disorders

Childhood Disorder	Intervention w/Empirical Support
Fears/phobias	Systematic desensitization
PTSD	Release play therapy
Aggression	Play group therapy
Adjustment reaction	Release play therapy
Oppositional	Parent-child interaction
ADHD	Cognitive-behavioral
Sexually abused	Abuse-specific play therapy
Selective mutism	Cognitive-behavioral
Anxiety	Cognitive-behavioral
OCD	Cognitive-behavioral
Obesity	Play group therapy
Reactive attachment	Theraplay/child-centered
Anger	Cognitive-behavioral
Chronic illness	Filial
Children of divorce	Play group therapy
Bereaved	Play group therapy
Children of alcoholics	Play group therapy
Foster/adoptive	Filial
Peer relationship	Play group therapy

Jennifer Lefebre, PsyD, RPT-S

I employ a developmental, attachment-based perspective in looking at a child's presenting competencies as well as within their struggles. I believe understanding the importance of attachment and neurobiology, particularly with our youngest clients who have suffered from trauma, is vital to our ability to have relationships with them and their families. My theoretical orientation is grounded in attachment theory (Bowlby, 1982, 1988), various neuroscience theories (Perry, 2009; Porges, 2004; Siegel, 1999; van der Kolk, 2014), and play therapy (Axline, 1969; Landreth, 2002; Schaefer & Drewes, 2014).

Siegel's *interpersonal neurobiology* and Porges's *polyvagal theory* combine well with Bowlby's *Attachment theory* in order to understand the connection between our bodies, minds, and the interplay within our relationships. The social engagement system is a playful mixture of activation and calming that helps us navigate these relationships. When combined with Perry's *neurosequential model* and van der Kolk's understanding of how trauma rewires the brain and affects the mind and body, we have a comprehensive approach to the child and family based on the core principles of neurodevelopment and traumatology.

Play promotes child development by building relationships, increasing social skills, developing empathetic connection, and building problem-solving capabilities (Landreth, 2002; Schaefer & Drewes, 2014). Children engage in play across cultures and play transcends language and ethnic barriers, allowing for the therapeutic powers of play to facilitate, initiate, and strengthen change.

I typically take a gradual, nondirective approach when possible, integrating evidence-based trauma and play therapies (i.e., Theraplay®, ARC, SMART, EMDR, and trauma-sensitive yoga) when needed.

Clair Mellenthin, MSW, RPT-S

I adhere to an integrated, systemic, prescriptive approach in my play therapy practice. My main theories of influence are attachment theory (Bowlby, 1969) and bioecological systems theory (Bronfenbrenner, 2005). I believe that it is critical that as clinicians, we take into account the environmental factors underlying a client's presenting problem and address the significant attachment relationships within each of the different systems. When we only look at a child as an individual and do not take into account their home environment, family and parental relationships, and other systems of influence, such as school, religious affiliation, culture, and community, we may be missing a huge component that needs to be addressed in treatment. I often tell my graduate students, "If you only focus on the presenting behavioral issues, you are going to miss the child".

Viewing treatment through the lens of attachment theory clarifies the underlying emotional and relational wounds that may be present in the emotional and/or behavioral issues that warranted a child's referral to treatment. Often, a child's acting out is a maladaptive attachment-seeking behavior or a response to an injured or ruptured attachment. I also believe wholeheartedly that involvement with the parents is a critical aspect of clinical care, as we can't expect the least powerful, most vulnerable members of the family system to be the one to create lasting change (Mellenthin, 2019). It is through repairing and strengthening the parent-child relationship that healing and change can take place.

I tend to utilize a prescriptive approach to each child's play therapy treatment, in order to tailor treatment to their specific treatment issues. Prescriptive play therapy allows for broad flexibility in practice, as it includes a variety of theories and interventions, that can be individualized to address the specific needs of the client (Schaefer & Drewes, 2016). Research (Chambless & Ollendick, 2001; Schaefer & Drewes, 2016) has shown that specific interventions work best for specific disorders and taking a cookie-cutter approach to humans has never been shown to work very well – we are too messy and complicated! By applying an integrated approach to play therapy, the clinician can pull from a variety of theories and techniques, blending them into a holistic treatment approach. I envision this as braiding – each strand a different theory, practice model, or technique blending together to create something beautiful and just the right fit for the child and family.

Akiko J. Ohnogi, PsyD

My primary play therapy theory is psychodynamic, which states that unconscious mental processes influence people's thoughts, feelings, and behavior. The significance and impact of early childhood relationships and experiences on later development are of important focus (Bromfield, 2003). As I believe that everyone is different, and every experience influences an individual, I utilize a prescriptive approach which tailors treatment interventions specifically for each individual (Ohnogi, 2013). The following is an example of how I utilized psychodynamic theory to conceptualize two cases and employed a prescriptive approach for treatment. This example addresses two eight-year-old children who were survivors of a tsunami in Thailand which killed many people.

Ben

"Ben" presented for treatment with his parents for separation anxiety concerns and various posttraumatic responses he was exhibiting. He appeared to have experienced a single trauma and was experiencing age-typical trauma symptoms. His attachment to his parents appeared stable. His parents demonstrated appropriate parenting styles and a reasonable understanding of child development.

Structured activities to regulate his autonomic nervous system were incorporated in the early stages of play therapy treatment. Ben readily utilized unstructured play. He often used the two sofas in the play therapy room to work on his fears and regain a feeling of safety. Additionally, a few unstructured parent-child play sessions were conducted to enhance their attachment and advance his feeling of protection. Parenting education was focused mainly on trauma reactions and neurological effects.

Meg

Meg's teacher referred her to play therapy treatment for attention, behavioral, emotional, and social difficulties which had worsened posttrauma. She had not received psychological treatment for a past car accident due to her parents thinking she would "get over it". In hindsight, they realized that her behavior had changed at the time. This realization, along with more current stressors, brought them to treatment.

I conceptualized Meg as a child with a history of unresolved trauma who had been retraumatized by her more current experience of a tsunami. Her attachment to her parents seemed unstable. She exhibited ambivalent behavior which could indicate that she was unable to rely on them.

Structured activities for regulation were incorporated throughout the initial sessions. Meg did not feel comfortable playing freely on her own, so as she became increasingly regulated, structured activities were introduced to address her emotions and cognitions. Structured activities with Meg and her parents were implemented to address attachment issues, and parenting education sessions regarding trauma, child development, and parenting skills were conducted.

Although these same-age children both experienced traumas, the interventions and level of parental support differed greatly. These differences included their relationships with and support from their parents, their individual personalities, their past histories, and their previous trauma experiences. In both cases, considering each child's distinct psychodynamics was important for conceptualizing and treating the underlying issues.

Mary Anne Peabody, EdD, RPT-S

I consider myself a prescriptive play therapist whereby my clinical decision-making includes individualized treatment of each client based on comprehensive assessments and the belief that some types of play therapy are more effective with certain disorders (Kaduson et al., 2020). This prescriptive approach involves triadic pairing of the client's presenting issues with the most efficacious treatment and the specific therapeutic change agent(s) that I am able to offer within the bounds of my training (Schaefer, 2018). Metaphorically, I envision my practice as a woven tapestry on a loom. The frame of the loom represents my firm belief in the therapeutic powers of play as the key drivers of the change process (Schaefer & Drewes, 2014). The horizontal threads that move back and forth, in and out, are the specific play therapy theories I have studied and received clinical supervision in using with clients. Still more threads include the specific client's circumstances and preferences, the presenting disorder or problem, cultural considerations, and current motivation and expectations of both the client and family (Norcross & Wampold, 2011; Schaefer, 2018). Final threads include my past experiences with a variety of clients, as well as my mistakes which humbly translate into some of my greatest lessons.

My initial training in play therapy theories began with cognitive behavioral (Knell, 2009) and Ecosystemic play therapy (O'Connor, 2015). Next, I received intense coursework in the humanistic child-centered play therapy theory (Landreth, 2012). Being early in my career, I conceptualized these seemingly disparate theories at opposite ends of a philosophical continuum, which is why I believe Adlerian play therapy (Kottman & Meany-Walen, 2016) was a welcomed discovery in my developmental training. I conceptualized Adlerian play therapy to fit somewhere in the middle of the continuum, synergistically and creatively complementing my own style, beliefs, and preferences. As my career matured, these theories became less dichotomous and I could readily acknowledge the many similarities between the theories, not just their differences. I accepted the strengths and limitations of the different orientations, which builds on why the concepts and principles of prescriptive play therapy align so well with me.

Prescriptive play therapy captures how I conceptualize decision-making in treatment and how I operationalize my actions. However, being prescriptive does not necessarily mean I am always integrative (Peabody & Schaefer, 2016).

I may practice under a single theory when I deem it sufficient to resolve the underlying cause of the client's problem. At other times, I may integrate one or more theories into a multifaceted approach to treat the range of complex psychological problems that the client is experiencing (Stricker & Gold, 2008). Reflecting back, my developmental journey followed what has been termed as an assimilative-integrative perspective (Kaduson et al., 2020; Messer, 1992), and my development is certainly continuing.

Dee Ray, PhD, RPT-S

My practice, teaching, and supervision of play therapy is driven by the belief that clinicians should be grounded in a theoretical orientation to play therapy. A counseling theory is an encompassing philosophy that proposes an understanding of human nature, personality development, and theory of change (Fall et al., 2017). When a play therapist matches their own personal belief system with a counseling theoretical orientation, this way of working guides their approach and plan with clients. I, personally, identify with person-centered theory (PCT; Rogers, 1942), the theoretical base for child-centered play therapy (CCPT). From a PCT theoretical perspective, persons are born with an actualizing tendency that, when provided the essential relational conditions, moves them toward the betterment of self, that, in turn, leads to social and emotional wellness (Ray, 2011). The organism of the person can be trusted to enhance the person and others in relationship with that person. It is only when a child encounters introjections from others or relational disruptions that the behaviors, cognitions, and emotions become separated from the internal system of wellness, resulting in incongruence between the child and the environment. In being able to clarify my belief system about how children come into the world and how they develop within the world, my role as a play therapist becomes clear. As a play therapist, I seek to provide the relational conditions necessary to facilitate the child's movement to connect with the internal organismic process that will allow them to move in the direction of congruence and health. Through the CCPT approach, I send a message of trust in the child, the message that they are worthy and capable of wellness, by providing an environment in which the child directs the process of play therapy. I follow the CCPT way-of-working because PCT matches my personal beliefs about humans and provides a consistent approach in the application of theory (Landreth, 2012; Ray, 2011), and my personal and professional experience has provided ample evidence of its effectiveness. Because CCPT is an actionable philosophy of working holistically with children, research over the last 80 years supports its effectiveness with children who demonstrate externalizing, internalizing, relational, academic, and social problems, as well as children who have experienced adverse childhood experiences or trauma (Bratton et al., 2005; Lin & Bratton, 2015; Ray et al., 2015).

Jessica Stone, PhD, RPT-S

I identify my psychological case conceptualization as a primarily nondirective, psychodynamic, and attachment-based theoretical foundation with a prescriptive play therapy approach. I believe early experiences teach each of us about the world, how people treat each other, how it is or is not acceptable for other people to treat us, what others define as our worth, and what our place is in the world. These young messages morph along the way through life by being challenged, supported, reinforced, and altered through each relationship a person experiences. When a client comes to me for services, I want to understand the answers to as many of the above questions as possible for that client. This informs me regarding their worldview. The modalities used with the client are approached prescriptively as "one size does not fit all" and would need to be tailored to the needs of the client. These modalities are also vetted prior to use to be certain that the therapeutic powers of play are activated (Schaefer & Drewes, 2014).

Daniel Sweeney, PhD, RPT-S

My primary approach to play therapy is essentially informed by my beliefs regarding the play therapy relationship and developmental fit. It is my opinion that regardless of theoretical or technical application, recognition of the importance of the play therapy relationship and developmental appropriateness is paramount. Having said this, I most closely align with Clark Moustakas's (1997) *Relationship Play Therapy*. Moustakas emphasizes that the therapist

> … waits for the child, serves the child with patience and dedication, until the child is ready to face issues and challenges of living in accordance with her or his own nature. Waiting expresses the therapist's faith in the child's powers to be and to grow. The child is regarded as a person of distinctiveness and integrity. Again and again, I saw that the relationship between child and therapist facilitates freedom of expression, that through the relationship the child discovers and affirms a real self.
>
> (Moustakas, 1997, p. 7)

For me, this focus on "waiting" and the relationship far outweighs all other factors, including the most intriguing techniques, regardless of the age of the play therapy client. This also eclipses the emphasis on the Schaefer and Drewes's therapeutic powers of play (Schaefer & Drewes, 2014). Whereas I largely endorse the therapeutic powers of play, I would contend that the "20 core agents of change" do not [indeed, *can* not] occur outside the development of a foundational therapeutic relationship.

Although my training and writing are reflective of a belief in child-centered play therapy [CCPT], I do not consider myself to be a child-centered play therapist. While I primarily use CCPT (Landreth, 2012) with young children, I do so for developmental reasons, more so than for theoretical reasons. I see this as a crucial distinctive. It is my perspective that many [perhaps a majority of] well-argued techniques are actually not a developmental fit for young children. I use play therapy with children because I believe that children lack the developmental, verbal, and cognitive sophistication that adults generally have. It seems therefore inconsistent to use a technique that fundamentally <u>requires</u> a verbal response. I have encountered numerous respected colleagues that have developed powerful play therapy techniques – that I would choose to use with preadolescents or adolescents rather than young children. For the sake of clarity, I define young children as children ranging from infancy through ten years old. I would encourage this book's readers to consider reviewing Dee Ray's book *A Therapist's Guide to Child Development* (2016).

All this to say that within a humanistic framework, I consider myself to be a relationship play therapist who primarily uses CCPT with young children. Across life span development, I use a variety of play/expressive therapy techniques, therefore being technically eclectic but theoretically consistent.

References

Ansbacher, H., & Ansbacher, R. (Eds.). (1956). *The individual psychology of Alfred Adler: A systematic presentation in selections from his writings.* Harper and Row.

Axline, V. M. (1969). *Play therapy.* Ballantine Books.

Bowlby, J. (1969). *Attachment.* Basic Books

Bowlby, J. (1982). *Attachment.* Basic Books.

Bowlby, J. (1988). *A secure base.* Basic Books.

Bratton, S., Ray, D., Rhine, T., & Jones, L. (2005). The efficacy of play therapy with children: A meta-analytic review of treatment outcomes. *Professional Psychology: Research and Practice, 36,* 376–390. doi:10.1037/0735-7028.36.4.376

Bromfield, R. (2003). Psychoanalytic play therapy. In C. E. Schaefer (Ed.), *Foundations of play therapy* (pp. 1–13). John Wiley & Sons, Inc.

Bronfenbrenner, U. (2005). *Making human beings human: The bioecological perspectives of human development.* Sage Publications.

Carlson, J., Watts, R., & Maniacci, M. (2005). *Adlerian therapy: Theory and practice.* American Psychological Association.

Chambless, D. L. & Ollendick, T. H. (2001). Empirically supported psychological interventions: Controversies and evidence. *Annual Review of Psychology, 52,* 685–716.

Drewes, A. A., Bratton, S. C., & Schaefer, C. E. (Eds.). (2011). *Integrative play therapy.* John Wiley & Sons Inc.

Fall, K., Holden, J., & Marquis, A. (2017). *Theoretical models of counseling and psychotherapy* (3rd ed.). Routledge.

Grant, R. J. (2017). *AutPlay therapy for children and adolescents on the autism spectrum: A behavioral play-based approach.* Routledge.

Kaduson, H. G., Cangelosi, D., & Schaefer, C. E. (Eds.). (1997). *The playing cure: Individualized play therapy for specific childhood problems.* Jason Aronson.

Kaduson, H. G., Cangelosi, D., & Schaefer, C. E. (Eds.). (2020). *Prescriptive play therapy: Tailoring interventions for specific childhood problems.* Guilford Press.

Kaduson, H. G., Schaefer, C. E. & Cangelosi, D. (2020). Basic principles and core practices of prescriptive play therapy. In H. G. Kaduson, D. Cangelosi, & C. E. Schaefer (Eds.), *Prescriptive play therapy: Tailoring interventions for specific childhood problems* (pp. 3–13). Guilford Press.

Knell, S. M. (2009). Cognitive behavioral play therapy: Theory and applications. In A. A. Drewes (Ed.), *Blending play therapy with cognitive behavioral therapy: Evidence-based and other effective treatments and techniques* (pp. 117–133). Wiley.

Kottman, T. (1999). Adlerian play therapy. *International Journal of Play Therapy, 10,* 1–12.

Kottman, T., & Meany-Walen, K. (2016). *Partners in play: An Adlerian approach to play therapy* (3rd ed.). American Counseling Association.

Landreth, G. L. (1991). *Play therapy: The art of the relationship.* Accelerated Development Inc. Publishers.

Landreth, G. L. (2002). *Play therapy: The art of the relationship* (2nd ed.). Routledge.

Landreth, G. L. (2012). *Play therapy: The art of the relationship* (3rd ed.). Brunner-Routledge.

Lin, Y., & Bratton, S. (2015). A meta-analytic review of child-centered play therapy approaches. *Journal of Counseling and Development, 93,* 45–58. 2147/10.1002/j.1556-6676.2015.00180.x

Mellenthin, C. (2019). *Attachment centered play therapy.* Routledge.

Messer, E. (1992). A critical examination of belief structures in integrative and eclectic psychotherapy. In J. C. Norcross & M. R. Goldfried (Eds.), *Handbook of psychotherapy integration* (2nd ed., pp. 130–165). Basic Books.

Moustakas, C. (1997). *Relationship play therapy.* Jason Aronson, Inc.

Norcross, J. C. (1991). Prescriptive matching in psychotherapy: An introduction. *Psychology, 28,* 439–443.

Norcross, J. C. & Wampold, B. F. (2011). What works for whom: Tailoring psychotherapy to the person. *Journal of Clinical Psychology in Session, 67*(2), 127–132.

O'Connor, K. J. (2015). Ecosystemic play therapy. In K. J. O'Connor, C. E. Schaefer, & L. D. Braverman (Eds.), *Handbook of play therapy* (2nd ed., pp. 195–226). Wiley.

Ohnogi, A. (2013). Creating safe space in play therapy with children. In H. Kotani & F. Bonds-White (Eds.), *Creating safe space through individual and group psychotherapy* (pp. 41–61). Institute of Psychoanalytic Systems Psychotherapy Press.

Peabody, M. A. & Schaefer, C. E. (2016). Towards semantic clarity in play therapy. *International Journal of Play Therapy, 25*(4), 197–202.

Perry, B. D. (2009). Examining child maltreatment through a neurodevelopmental lens: Clinical application of the neurosequential model of therapeutics. *Journal of Loss and Trauma, 14,* 240–255. doi:10.1080/15325020903004350

Porges, S. W. (2004). Neuroception: A subconscious system for detecting threats and safety. *Zero to Three, 24*(5), 19–24.

Ray, D. (2011). *Advanced play therapy: Essential conditions, knowledge, and skills for child practice.* Routledge.

Ray, D., Armstrong, S., Balkin, R., & Jayne, K. (2015). Child centered play therapy in the schools: Review and meta-analysis. *Psychology in the Schools, 52,* 107–123.

Rogers, C. (1942). *Counseling and psychotherapy.* Houghton Mifflin Company.

Schaefer, C. E. (2018, December). The 10 basic principles of prescriptive play therapy. *Play Therapy, 13*(4), 24–27.

Schaefer, C. E. & Drewes, A. A. (Eds.). (2014). *The therapeutic powers of play: 20 core agents of change* (2nd ed.). John Wiley & Sons.

Schaefer, C. E. & Drewes, A. A. (2016). Prescriptive play therapy. In K. J. O'Connor, C._E. Schaefer, & L. D. Braverman (Eds.), *Handbook of play therapy* (2nd ed., pp. 227–240). Wiley.

Siegel, D. J. (1999). *The developing mind: Toward a neurobiology of interpersonal experience.* Guilford Press.

Stricker, G., & Gold, J. (2008). Integrative psychotherapy. In J. L. Lebow (Ed.), *Twenty-first century psychotherapies: Contemporary approaches to theory and practice* (pp. 389–423). Wiley & Sons.

van der Kolk, B. A. (2014). *The body keeps the score: Brain, mind, and body in the healing of trauma.* Viking.

VanFleet, R. (2014). *Filial therapy: strengthening parent-child relationships through play* (3rd ed.). Professional Resource Press.

2 What Advice Would You Give Someone Just Getting Started in Play Therapy?

Jeff Ashby, PhD, RPT-S

In considering my therapeutic work with children, Kurt Lewin's (1951) famous maxim, "There is nothing so practical as a good theory" (p. 169) rings true. My primary advice for someone just beginning play therapy is twofold. First, identify and cultivate a theoretical perspective for your work. It is very easy to become enamored of specific techniques (I know because I have certainly done it!) and then think about where they might be helpful with clients, without a clear rationale in the context of a treatment plan or broader theoretical conceptualization. Without a solid theoretical base for one's play therapy, one may default to an indiscriminate "mish-mash of theories, a hugger-mugger of procedures, a gallimaufry of therapies, having no proper rationale or empirical verification" (Eysenck, 1970, p. 145). While systematic eclecticism may be a viable approach, it is "the product of years of painstaking clinical research and experience" (Norcross & Goldfried, 2003, p. 20) and, as a result, not the best approach for those starting in play therapy. Adopting a prominent theory of play therapy (e.g., child-centered, cognitive-behavioral, psychoanalytic, Gestalt, or even Adlerian) gives the beginning play therapist a set of guidelines to predict, explain, and structure interventions. Consistently using a theory of play therapy also allows the play therapist a place to which they can return when they are struggling with clients (rather than simply casting around for a new/different technique).

The second piece of advice I would offer the beginning play therapist is to pursue the advanced credential of Registered Play Therapist (RPT), a credential granted by the Association for Play Therapy (www.a4pt.org). The Credentialing Standards for the Registered Play Therapist (APT, 2019a) lay out a groundwork for the systematic development of competence and expertise in play therapy. I would recommend that the beginning play therapist follow these guidelines (outlined in three phases and including play therapy instruction, clinical practice, and supervision). In addition to offering a roadmap for the development of competence/expertise, pursuing the RPT will bring the beginning play therapist into the community of play therapists through attending trainings and receiving supervision. The collegial interaction and peer consultation that happen naturally in the context of the play therapy community (e.g., attending the APT annual meeting) are, for me, an important means by which I have continued to develop in my play therapy practice – and I would recommend it to the beginning play therapist.

Robert Jason Grant, EdD, RPT-S

It is a journey, not a destination. I think it's important to enjoy the process of learning about play therapy and growing as a skilled play therapist. I also believe this is a lifelong commitment. There is always something more to learn, always more growth that can happen. My beginnings as a play therapist were a bit disjointed. I did not have any play therapy courses in my master's program. I began taking play therapy trainings after I graduated with my master's degree. Early in my career, there were few play therapy trainings offered and I often traveled to receive training. The training was not always very streamlined as I often took trainings when and where I could get them. Luckily, I had very good supervision. I was working in a mental health clinic surrounded by other professionals who were doing play therapy, so I had a rich environment of supervision, both formal and informal, and a lot of opportunity for consultation. My clinical environment exposed me to many play therapy theories and ideas and gave me the opportunity to explore and implement what I was learning in trainings.

The weaving together of learning, practical implementation with clients, and supervision is critical. Those beginning in play therapy should strive to weave together this balance. I would encourage individuals to pursue the Registered Play Therapist (RPT) credential. This credential is recognized and overseen by the Association for Play Therapy (APT). It identifies an individual as having obtained a level of training in play therapy (recognized by APT), completed numerous hours in clinical application with clients, and completed many hours of supervision with a Registered Play Therapist-Supervisor (RPT-S). Getting involved with APT can also be important for those beginning in play therapy. The national organization governs many things related to play therapy and can serve as a valuable resource for those learning about play therapy.

There are many paths that someone can take in pursuing play therapy. One person's journey will look differently than another person. It is important to remember that no matter what your path looks like, make the most of the journey and enjoy learning about and experiencing play therapy work. Children and families need more play therapists; this is important work we are doing, and we are often working with our most vulnerable populations. As you are on the journey of pursuing play therapy, make the most of learning opportunities, acquire quality formal and informal supervision and consultation, learn proper self-care, and enjoy the experience of becoming a play therapist.

Heidi Gerard Kaduson, PhD, RPT-S

Play therapy has been used for over 50 years, and there are so many different approaches at this time. Therefore, I would advise that each person who is beginning to use play therapy receive training from approved providers in different perspectives and theories. By doing so, the therapist can find which theoretical approach is best suited for the therapist to use as their foundational theoretical approach.

It is very important for all therapists to continue to learn and receive approved training throughout their career. There is always something more to learn. To ensure that play therapists are able to obtain high-quality continuing education, the Association for Play Therapy has established standards for Approved Providers of Play Therapy Continuing Education (Association for Play Therapy, 2019b). However, quality education is not enough. Play therapists will benefit from participating in their own personal therapy as well. Working with children can easily trigger someone's early past, which might negatively reflect in their work with children. This must be understood before practicing play therapy with clients. For the safety of both the therapist and the child, the therapist should be in his or her own psychotherapy. In addition, play therapists need to find Registered Play Therapist-Supervisors to receive the proper supervision while they work with children of all ages. The supervision has two main functions:

1   *Education*: to provide a regular space for the supervisee to reflect on content and process of their work, help relate theory to practice, to give an opportunity to think and develop ideas, and to develop understanding and skills within the work
2   *Support*: to be validated as a person and therapist, to give constructive positive and critical feedback, to keep play therapists accountable for the monitoring and quality of the work being done with the children, and to utilize the personal and professional resources of supervision)

By being appropriately supervised and educated while working with children, the play therapist will develop and grow whether they choose to become a Registered Play Therapist and then a Registered Play Therapist-Supervisor or not. Play therapists can learn a great deal from the children they treat as well as from peers and authorities in the field. Being open to learning more is an important step in becoming a true play therapist.

Jennifer Lefebre, PsyD, RPT-S

I would recommend attending a play therapy conference, listening to a variety of speakers, and meeting people in the field. There are so many approaches and styles, and a conference is an excellent way to get a sampling of diversity within the field of play therapy. If a conference is not an option, there are many web-based podcasts or interviews where aspiring play therapists can get exposure to a variety of topics and presenters in the field. I believe it is important to know a little bit about a variety of topics in play therapy – as many as you can! Understanding a variety of play therapy topics creates a well-rounded play therapist and is also part of earning a registered play therapist credential. Developing an area of specialization as a play therapist is very rewarding as well. To be able to learn as much as you can and grow into an expert in a certain diagnostic category, developmental age group, or type of play therapy provides an area of competency for the play therapist to feel grounded and self-assured.

Lastly, finding a supervisor who matches your personality and interests is also very important, arguably the most important part of the process. The supervision process is something that really should not be overlooked or minimized in becoming a solid play therapist. I recommend that my students seek supervisors not based on location but based on skill set and interests. For example, I treat complex trauma – if a supervisee wants to work solely with learning challenges in a school system, I would not be a good match, whereas a school-based play therapist-supervisor would meet their needs in a more direct, applicable, and well-rounded manner.

Clair Mellenthin, MSW, RPT-S

My first piece of advice is to find a good play therapy supervisor and mentor to help you on your journey to becoming a confident and competent play therapist. It is so important to have supervision throughout your professional life, no matter how green or seasoned you may be. I am grateful to have supervisors, mentors, friends, and colleagues in the play therapy community whom I regularly consult with regarding difficult cases and issues of countertransference and transference, and as I learn new practice models and/or theories.

My second piece of advice is to become grounded in theory. It is so important to have a strong theoretical foundation to stand on as a clinician. Learn and be trained in the different theoretical models of play therapy. Then seek out in-depth learning and training into a specific model initially to develop a sense of competence. Find what speaks to you and where you feel most comfortable and then research, read, get trained, and use it. If you are just using different techniques you pull from a book without an understanding of the theoretical framework and possible ramifications, you may unintentionally cause real harm in your work with a client. Techniques are not play therapy; they are just a component of a play therapy approach or model.

My last piece of advice is to seek out and become a credentialed Registered Play Therapist (RPT) from the Association for Play Therapy (www.a4pt.org) or its equivalent if outside the United States. Join the Play Therapy Association in your home country or place of employment. This not only provides you with a roadmap of how to seek out qualified trainings, research, and resources but also will involve you in a network of like-minded and passionate play therapists. Attend continuing education workshops and conferences, read new and classic play therapy literature, and continue learning and developing therapeutic skills and knowledge well into your career. This will help you become a confident, *competent* play therapist!

Akiko J. Ohnogi, PsyD

Of the many things that I would like to advise someone just getting started in play therapy, the first one would be to enjoy what you are doing. Treating someone who is suffering emotionally is an immense responsibility and must be taken seriously. I believe that in order to be able to do this kind of work effectively, the play therapist must enjoy their profession. This enjoyment helps to counteract the potential burdens and any negativity they may encounter during the treatment process.

Having a solid foundation in play therapy theory will contribute to the therapist's level of enjoyment. When you have just started as a play therapist, you may want to base your treatment of clients on a single theory. Focusing on a theory you have studied and which feels comfortable will lead to a solid foundation. It is important to keep an open mind to other theories and approaches, and attend trainings to expand your understanding so that you can find one that fits you well. Never try to conduct play therapy if you do not have a theory on which to base your treatment.

Continuing to learn about play therapy by attending workshops and conferences and keeping up with research will contribute to therapist comfort. Areas of interest can include play therapy, play, child development, parenting, diagnosis, treatment, and more. Additionally, for best treatment planning and implementing, a play therapist should also have a basic understanding of neurobiology and how play therapy affects the brain.

Novice play therapists (and in my belief all play therapists), should receive supervision, preferably from a play therapy supervisor who can incorporate play and activities as part of the supervision. Not only will supervision support the actual conceptualization and treatment of a case, but it will be an integral part of your own personal support in growth and maintenance of you as a professional play therapist.

It is always important that you aspire toward a balance of appropriately challenging yourself while ensuring you are within your ethical scope of ability regarding the treatment that you are providing. You do not want to become overwhelmed by taking on difficult or complex cases without access to appropriate support.

Always, always, always remember to incorporate self-care into your daily life. Professionals in the caring business have the highest risk of burning out because they have a tendency to place other's needs before their own. Mental health professionals also seem to have the tendency to think that they are "immune" to whatever ails their clients. Remember that you need to take care of yourself in order to be able to help others effectively.

Lastly, remember that you are a professional. You most likely know much more about child development, mental health, play, and play therapy than the average person. Feel confident and show it, while remembering that there is always room for growth.

Mary Anne Peabody, EdD, RPT-S

I was fortunate to be a student of play studies before becoming a play therapist. My career began in the fields of child life and recreational therapy, and I worked for many years in children's hospitals. This foundational start allowed me to study child development, family studies, and play prior to learning play therapy theories. At the time, I did not realize what a benefit this would offer me as a future play therapist. Accordingly, I strongly advocate that beginning play therapists study child development, then move into a comprehensive study of the therapeutic powers of play prior to learning specific play therapy theories or techniques (Peabody & Schaefer, 2019). This stance aligns with advice to concentrate on learning and practicing one play therapy theory extremely well under the clinical supervision of a Registered Play Therapist-Supervisor. I believe the supervisor needs to observe multiple play sessions of the supervisee with multiple clients and offer substantial feedback. I suggest to deeply study and practice within one or two theoretical orientations early in your career, trying to avoid the lure of becoming certified in many different approaches. Realize as a licensed mental health professional in an ever-expanding field, you have a professional lifetime to keep learning and growing. Go for quality versus quantity.

If accessible, I strongly encourage university level courses over workshop trainings, as university coursework typically involves session recordings and transcript analysis based on theoretical conceptualization, supervision, additional readings, and scholarly papers. I believe it is foundational to becoming a clinically sound play therapist. Individuals in workshop trainings rarely engage in this level of intense study. Having said this, I am aware some certification programs require educational assignments, observations of practice, and supervision requirements that are spread out under the supervision of a registered play therapy supervisor. These experiences would certainly be similar to university level training and address the need for practitioners to continue to develop their play therapy skills without access to higher education coursework.

Other advice I have is to continue to be supervised by a registered play therapy supervisor (RPT-S) or participate in a consultation group with other registered play therapists throughout your practice career. Additionally, if possible, join the play therapy professional association located within the country or region in which you practice. This type of professional membership allows access to the most current information, research, and trends in the play therapy field. Furthermore, always remain a student by continually reading both practice and research articles. And above all, stay curious.

Dee Ray, PhD, RPT-S

My most frequent advice to new play therapists is to seek solid education and supervision in child development and play therapy. For me, solid training is signified by the qualifications of the trainer, the depth and accuracy of the content, and attention to the reflective process of education. First, teachers/presenters/trainers in play therapy should be well-versed in the history, process, and research of play therapy. An effective play therapy teacher is well-read and familiar with multiple approaches to play therapy, even if they subscribe to one approach over others. The teacher is able to ground educational content to actual research (i.e., not repeat what they read from someone's opinion but actual data to support content). The depth and accuracy of play therapy curriculum content is marked by the provision of rationale for play therapy processes and actions. Content is rooted in a theoretically based foundation, research, and descriptive relational processes.

Often, play therapy training content involves the delivery of multiple activities or techniques that are untethered to purpose, intentionality, or therapeutic processing of such activities. I find these types of trainings to be meaningless at best, and dangerous, at worst, in cases when participants take the latest technique to a play therapy session without any real knowledge or consideration of how and why it is being used. The reflective process of education is as critical a component of training as any provision of content. Solid play therapy training involves the personal reflection of the play therapist regarding their belief systems, their values, their participation in play therapy approaches/techniques as clients, and their readiness to engage in play therapy processes. When I hear play therapists ask questions or post on social media, the most likely reason for questions appears to be lack of training. Finding good training can be difficult and costly, but ultimately, when play therapists take the time, energy, and resources to participate in solid training, the sacrifices are worthwhile as demonstrated through their increase in competence, confidence, and treatment outcomes.

Second, and just as important, new play therapists need the mentorship of a qualified play therapist-supervisor. Although credentials, such as Registered Play Therapist-Supervisor (RPT-S; Association for Play Therapy, 2019b) are notable, new play therapists should seek supervisors who are knowledgeable and grounded in play therapy processes, establish relationships in which the supervisee is safe to ask and process the tough questions, and provide feedback and guidance on play therapy and the course of becoming a play therapist. Even experienced mental health professionals should seek supervision when they are becoming play therapists as the process of play therapy is unique from other counseling modalities. So, my best advice is to find qualified educators and supervisors.

Jessica Stone, Ph.D., RPT-S

Have a solid foundation in theory. Explore many different theories, notice what the differences and the commonalities are, and discover what components fit with your integrity, personality, and beliefs about change, cure, and goals. It is critical that a play therapist deeply understand the answers to the "why, what, where, when, who, and how" questions regarding play therapy treatment.

A play therapist must be solid in the play therapy fundamentals and flexible in their application– OR – if one is a purist, know your approach is x and understand the benefits and limitations. If the treatment is not appropriate for a client, be sure to refer responsibly. There is no "one size fits all" in play therapy.

It is important to know how to frontload conversations with parents, caregivers, and collateral contacts to ensure informed consent and open, thorough communication. The therapist who has explored the why, what, where, when, who, and how questions can have a solid, rich conversation with others. The strength and confidence that comes with understanding the play therapy approach, and one's position within it, will breed confidence in others as well.

The items in the playroom should be thoughtfully chosen and familiar. Use the item and know it well. The goal is to be so familiar with the item that the focus during the use is on the process of the therapeutic interaction, etc. and not the mechanics of the use. The comfort and knowledge the therapist has regarding the items in the playroom will contribute to the overall ease, safety, and confidence of the client, the family, and the therapist. A play therapist could ask questions such as: what does this item contribute to the room? The client? The therapeutic process? Is it congruent with the theoretical foundation? What does the use of this item contribute to the understanding of the client? The ability to reach the therapeutic goals? Etc. Other questions regarding play therapy room items is regarding set-up. Does the arrangement of items portray the message or therapeutic environment desired? How can the space be altered to convey the desired underlying dynamic?

Finally, always seek knowledge. Never underestimate the power of perspective. Be sure to include self-care in your life. Seek new challenges but maintain healthy boundaries. Know yourself and your work as best you can and continue to know each more thoroughly with every year in your career.

Daniel Sweeney, Ph.D., RPT-S

Initially, I would say that my advice for new play therapists would be the same as for therapists planning to specialize in any area in mental health: that would be to recognize that it is crucial to be a well-trained general mental health practitioner before being a specialist. A solid foundation is necessary before any specialization can occur.

In addition to this, there are several [somewhat philosophical] things that I believe new play therapists need to remember:

- Always be hopeful. The play therapist should be a lender of hope for children and parents that often have little to no hope. If we can have hope for them, we have already made a big step toward any goal.

- When you lack confidence with any given client, don't despair – you are simply human. When you lack confidence in self, have confidence in the process. The therapy process works. Play therapy works.
- Never stop seeking help. The best and most experienced play therapists continue to consult. If you ever get to the point of thinking you have all of the answers, you've moved from confidence to over-confidence – which is another word for arrogance.
- Be genuine. Be faithful to your instincts, your theory, and yourself. Genuineness is instantly recognizable – to children and their parents, to your colleagues, and to your family and friends.
- Be willing to make mistakes, and to learn from them. The ability to overcome our mistakes speaks to our own resiliency. Play therapists can't expect resiliency from our clients if we have none.
- Practice what you preach in terms of self-care. It's possible that our clients will only get as "healthy" as we promote the same principles of health within ourselves. We simply cannot give drinks from a well that is empty.
- We may need to "get out of the way". It's not just a CCPT concept that clients have within themselves the resources to heal when provided with therapeutic conditions. Play therapists, like all psychotherapists, have the privilege to join hurt children on difficult journeys. Walking this path does not always mean the therapist takes control of the process.
- Never forget the importance of the playroom being a "free and protected" space. This involves the Jungian concept of *temenos* (Jung, 1977): that the therapy room and process – and the playroom itself – provide a boundary between the sacred and the profane. Children must believe they are fully safe – emotionally, psychologically, spiritually, and physically.

References

Association for Play Therapy (1997). *History speaks: Frey interview*. http://youtu.be/6cxO0UQZFuo.

Association for Play Therapy (2019a). https://www.a4pt.org/page/CredentialsHomepage.

Association for Play Therapy (2019b). Credentialing standards for the Registered Play Therapist: APT professional credentialing program. https://cdn.ymaws.com/www.a4pt.org/resource/resmgr/credentials/2020_credentials/rpt_stand_22aug2019.pdf.

Eysenck, H. J. (1970). *The structure of human personality* (3rd ed.). Methuen.

Jung, C. G. (1977). *Symbols of transformation*. Princeton University Press.

Lewin, K. (1951). *Field theory in social science: Selected theoretical papers* (D. Cartwright, Ed). Harper & Row.

Norcross, J. C., & Goldfried, M. R. (2003). *Handbook of psychotherapy integration*. Oxford University Press

Peabody, M. A., & Schaefer, C. E. (2019). The therapeutic powers of play: The heart and soul of play therapy. *Play Therapy, 14*(3), 4–6.

3 What Are the Key Characteristics of a Well-Trained Play Therapist?

Jeff Ashby, PhD, RPT-S

In their explication of the process of becoming an RPT, APT outlines 18 specific competencies as "essential to the competent practice of play therapy" (APT, 2019; p. 12). These competencies are organized into areas of Knowledge & Understanding of Play Therapy, Clinical Play Therapy Skills, and Professional Engagement. They appropriately identify key competencies including understanding child development, having the ability to conceptualize play therapy cases through a theoretical lens, and demonstrating ethical engagement in practice. Certainly, these 18 competencies are critical when one considers the "key characteristics of a well-trained play therapist".

Another, more broadly conceptualized, set of characteristics that are important to the play therapist can be aptly borrowed from the multicultural counseling literature (e.g., Sue, 1998). It is appropriate to view play therapist's key characteristics from this lens because, as Pederson (1990) aptly noted, "all mental health counselling is multicultural" (p. 94). Sue (1998) conceptualized multicultural counseling as comprising three component parts: awareness, knowledge, and skills. I believe these three components are key characteristics of well-trained play therapists. Knowledge would include the competencies listed in the APT Credentialing Standards (APT, 2019) but also include an understanding of the worldviews of clients and the influence of racism/oppression and social and cultural factors. Similarly, skills would include the competencies listed in the APT standards but also the ability to tailor interventions to clients. While knowledge and skills are extremely important, I would highlight awareness as a particularly important characteristic for the well-trained play therapist. Awareness involves a play therapist's self-understanding, openness to supervision and consultation, acknowledgement of personal issues that may impact their work in play therapy (e.g., countertransference), and the understanding of one's own culture, values, and potential biases in their work. I believe that the characteristic of awareness leads play therapists to ongoing self-exploration, consultation, and even supervision, deepening their expertise in play therapy practice. The play therapists I admire most are characterized by this sense of awareness and, as a result, are always learning and growing.

Robert Jason Grant, EdD, RPT-S

A well-trained play therapist should first be knowledgeable in counseling and psychological theory and practice – they should possess basic therapeutic skills such as unconditional positive regard for the client, empathy, and a non-judgmental attitude. They should also be knowledgeable in child growth and development – a working knowledge in child development processes and stages. Beyond these two foundational child mental health constructs, a play therapist should be knowledgeable in one or more seminal play therapy theories and well trained in theories and approaches for the populations they are working with. A well-trained play therapist has also received proper and meaningful supervision and continues to seek out supervision and/or consultation as needed. Supervision should be obtained in the beginning of learning play therapy, especially when pursuing a play therapy credential, and supervision should continue in formal or informal ways throughout the play therapist's career.

I believe a well-trained play therapist always understands there is more they can learn. There should be a commitment to meaningful continuing education. This process should not be an activity to check off a credential requirement. Play therapists should continually be pursuing learning and education to increase their knowledge, skill set, and stay aware of research. There should be an understanding of ethical guidelines and an awareness of the therapeutic powers of play. Learning and education about play therapy should manifest in purposeful application. Well trained play therapists will know how to synthesize learning and clinical implementation.

I also believe that the well-trained play therapist enjoys working with children and families, and finds the process of play therapy valuable and meaningful. Through the years of implementing play therapy, and training and speaking about play therapy, the joy of doing and teaching play therapy has never dimmed. I cannot imagine doing anything else, and I cannot imagine working with children and not implementing play therapy. I see this same passion in several well-trained play therapists I have known. There is a love for play therapy and fierceness in protecting and promoting the integrity of play therapy.

Heidi Gerard Kaduson, PhD, RPT-S

I believe that all well-trained play therapists should first and foremost believe in the therapeutic powers of play. They also need to know the stages and developmental theories of children and play, how play is a therapeutic metaphor which should be understood and processed with their supervisors and have a knowledge of child development and normal developmental processes. I think it is imperative that all of us have the ability to critically evaluate a range of theoretical frameworks and therapeutic approaches other than play therapy in order to be able to give the best treatment possible, as well as understand the dynamics of the family relationship that impact the child. This includes understanding the culture in which the child lives, as well as traditions and feelings toward psychotherapy of any kind. In addition, one should know the full process of play therapy, such as assessment, evaluation, collaboration with family members and others, and how play therapy may impact the child and all other support systems. Certain key issues that are relevant to all children have to do with culture and traditions of different families.

Knowledge of a child's physical, cultural, social, emotional, religious, and cognitive development is necessary to treat each individual child. All of these aspects will impact the child and the play therapy treatment. We need training to continue as we treat children, since changes even in the environment, climate, and political areas can contribute to children's difficulties. Since trauma and attachment are key areas of psychological disturbances, the impact of these issues need to be understood and assessed. In addition, as new research reveals more controversial information regarding cause, correlation or effects, play therapists need to be constantly aware of new interest research, which may assist in the treatment of their child client.

Lastly, I believe that all play therapists need to be aware of childhood diseases and disorders. We may be the only people who spend 30–45 minutes face to face with a child in play, which will reveal more than any question and answer interview or inventory you can do. A well-trained play therapist should be open to new information, reviewing research, be involved with all the ecosystems of the child, and be willing to act as an advocate for any child that is being treated (O'Connor, 2016). Finally, a well-trained play therapist should be grounded in a theoretical approach and be familiar with other theoretical approaches so that they are flexible enough to decide what theoretical approach is needed for the child and to implement techniques from the therapeutic powers of play.

Jennifer Lefebre, PsyD, RPT-S

Play therapy truly is "the art of the relationship" Garry Landreth (2002). Children need adults in their lives who are compassionate, good listeners, gentle, and creative. Flexibility, open mindedness, and playfulness (of course!) are also essential to the success of a well-trained play therapist. Siegel and Bryson (2011) discuss how children need to be perceived deeply and empathically (seen), assisted with their difficult emotions and situations (soothed), and kept safe and secure. Play therapists should hold these characteristics in the highest regard.

With that being said, I believe self-awareness – an understanding of who you are as a person and within the therapeutic relationship (both inside and outside of the play therapy room) – is a priority for a well-trained play therapist. Knowledge of your own limits and boundaries, as well as your strengths and areas to grow, should be explored and understood. As play therapists, we feel empathy, get triggered by traumatogenic materials, and have our own histories. Transference is common in the play therapy relationship, especially since we are the container for our clients' most challenging materials. As a trauma therapist, I engage in very deep work with my clients, and I often say my shadow comes out to play with the shadows of the children I work with. Counter-transference is often mentioned in trainings, but it is not often thoroughly understood or discussed. I believe an awareness of our own shadows, all of the parts and the pieces within us that get activated in these moments, is vital for the work play therapists do. As such, self-awareness and supervision allow us to reflect on the deeper meanings within the session, and to recognize and embrace the parts within ourselves that make us who we are as therapist and people.

Clair Mellenthin, MSW, RPT-S

I believe the key characteristics of a well-trained play therapist are similar to those who have qualified to be credentialed as a Registered Play Therapist (RPT) from the Association for Play Therapy (APT) or its equivalent in other countries, such as the Registered Qualified Play Therapist from the British Association of Play Therapists (BAPT). These therapists are required to hold a master's or higher clinical mental health degree in one of the following disciplines: counseling, marriage and family therapy, psychiatry, psychology, or social work with demonstrated coursework in child development, theories of personality, principles of psychotherapy, child and adolescent psychopathology, and ethics (APT, 2019, p. 6). This ensures that as a student, they have had several years of schooling and scholarly development in critical theoretical components, as well as have participated in supervised clinical internships and professional development within their scope of a mental health degree. In addition, these play therapists accumulate years of training and continuing education (150+) hours focused specifically on play therapy theoretical concepts, application, and practice, as well as supervised postgraduate clinical play therapy experience from an experienced Registered Play Therapist-Supervisor (RPT-S) (APT, 2019).

In addition to their theoretical knowledge, foundation, and application, I believe other characteristics of a well-trained play therapist include a willingness to ask for help and support, an ability to identify their own feelings of transference and countertransference, and a willingness to and desire to continue their learning and development regardless of their years of experience and training. They should also have a mentor in the field of play therapy that they can consult for support, advice, and encouragement, as well as help navigating and strengthening their own professional development. These well-trained clinicians are also working with, supervising, and teaching new and fellow play therapists, helping to train the next generation of clinicians.

Akiko J. Ohnogi, PsyD

I believe that one can keep learning throughout life. It is necessary for all professionals to continue studying regardless of how advanced or well-known they are in their field. With this in mind, I believe that a well-trained play therapist will have the following characteristics at all the various stages of their profession, whether it be a novice just having graduated from graduate school, or one who has been in the field for decades.

A well-trained play therapist has:

1   a vast and deep knowledge of play therapy theories, keeps up with current research on play therapy, development, various psychological disorders, treatment effects of various interventions, play, and so on, and a basic understanding of how the brain works and the effects play therapy interventions have on it.

2   knowledge regarding the appropriate use of techniques that are correspond with the underlying theory the play therapist is utilizing, as well as any research which supports the treatment effects of those interventions.

3   the flexibility to adjust and "prescribe" the best treatment in a manner that results in the client feeling supported.

4   a focus on being attuned to the child's parents, colleagues, staff, other professionals, and one's own feelings, along with being able to respond, react, interact, and behave accordingly.

5   awareness of any transference and countertransference at all times, from and toward children and their parents. Other professionals with whom you liaison may also be a trigger for the clients, the other professional, and/or yourself. Making sure that you use any transferences therapeutically and deal with your feelings of countertransference outside of the sessions with your client is a must.

6   confidence in being a well-educated, trained, humble professional who has expertise and successes in treatment and an openness to new possibilities.

7   self-awareness which includes knowing one's own limits. Do not try to take on more than you can handle or treat issues which are outside your scope of practice and/or knowledge.

8   an ability to acknowledge that the play therapist is human. Daily life will affect a therapist as a person and inevitably as a clinician. If, for example, your mother is very sick and you are very worried, you are anxious being pregnant with your first child, or you are super excited about your first-year wedding anniversary, be aware that these emotions will affect how you conduct sessions.

9   a focus of incorporating self-care into daily life. Be able to ask for support, including your own psychological treatment if/when necessary.

Mary Anne Peabody, EdD, RPT-S

I believe a key characteristic of a well-trained play therapist is a willingness to become a master of their craft. This involves a commitment to lifelong professional development that includes conceptual, informational, and relational competencies. The conceptual includes a strong educational foundation in child development and the therapeutic powers of play, prior to learning seminal and historically significant play therapy theories (Peabody & Schaefer, 2019). Conceptually, a play therapist needs an understanding of cultural considerations, bio-ecological influences or systems theory, and the intersection of trauma, attachment, neuroscience, social and emotional wellness. Next a well-trained play therapist should have informational knowledge about evidence-based practices for specific disorders commonly addressed in play therapy clients (Schaefer, 2018) and basic play therapy terminology (Peabody & Schaefer, 2016).

As a general mental health provider, informational knowledge should also exist in topical areas such as understanding psychopathology across the life span, general mental health diagnosis, treatment planning, and an array of valid and reliable assessment measures to inform treatment decisions. Additionally, a well-trained play therapist would have informational knowledge of the ethical, legal, and confidentiality issues surrounding treating minors, and an understanding of the standards of their particular mental health license.

In terms of relational skill sets, a well-trained play therapist would know how to build therapeutic alliances with families and children. They would have strong verbal, nonverbal, and written communication skills. They should also possess well developed consultation skills to address the collateral needs inherent in a play therapy practice and welcome strong parent/ caregiver involvement in the treatment of children. Another skill set includes accepting and welcoming feedback through the iterative process of reflective practice and supervision. Included in this reflective practice should be an examination of a therapist's own playfulness and a willingness to continue to stay playful within their own professional growth. Clearly, the developmental nature of becoming a play therapist is a continual process of growth that requires clinical supervision, professional development, mistake making, patience, reflective practice, and experience. The process cannot and should not be rushed.

Dee Ray, PhD, RPT-S

A well-trained play therapist is a person who is knowledgeable, skillful, and possesses the personal characteristics necessary to provide essential conditions of therapy. Regarding knowledge, the well-trained play therapist operates within a consistent theoretical orientation from which the therapist conceptualizes the child and the child's struggles. The conceptualization process leads to a coherent plan for treatment that corresponds to the child's needs. Additionally, a play therapist's knowledge base ideally includes familiarity with child development theories, history and role of play in child development, medical knowledge relevant to children, criteria for diagnostic categories, role of psychopharmacological drugs for children, etiology and symptoms of typical presenting problems, current educational methods used in local schools, popular parenting methods, current scholarly research on child mental health, and basic research knowledge used to critically analyze literature (Ray, 2011). In order to acquire this breadth and depth of knowledge, a key personal characteristic of a well-trained play therapist is the desire and motivation to learn and to continue to learn over a professional lifetime.

Personal characteristics are critically fundamental and set the course to becoming a well-trained play therapist. The basics of building a play therapy relationship with a child involve the therapist's ability to provide empathic understanding and unconditional positive regard in a genuine manner (Rogers, 1957). Empathic understanding requires play therapists to take on the child's worldview, attempting to fully know the child's thoughts and feelings, and how they work together to result in behaviors. The empathic play therapist is curious about the inner dynamics of the child, open to seeing the world as the child does, and yet holds boundaries between self and other so as not to become enmeshed in the child's world. In working with children who have experienced extensive and multiple traumas, I may struggle with holding empathic understanding with a child because of the toll it takes on me to experience the pain and hurt that the child has experienced. Yet the experience and communication of empathic understanding is essential to the healing relationship.

Second, I believe that experiencing unconditional positive regard for the child is another essential feature of the healing therapeutic relationship. Unconditional positive regard includes warm acceptance of the child (Rogers, 1957), prizing the child, and believing in the capability of the child. The therapist's ability to hold unconditional positive regard is often tested when working with challenging children. Well-trained play therapists operate with awareness of their level of unconditional positive regard for each child and a desire to increase regard when they are struggling in a therapeutic relationship. Finally, another key characteristic of a well-trained play therapist is the movement and aspiration to work from a genuine and authentic way-of-being. The effective play therapist seeks to have a high level of awareness, allows awareness to be integrated into the self-concept, and demonstrates a willingness to be appropriately transparent in their process of congruence.

Jessica Stone, PhD, RPT-S

A well-trained play therapist will have a solid, well thought through theoretical foundation which is reevaluated and formulated throughout their career. They will continuously seek knowledge and be open to new concepts, implement self-care, know one's self well enough to place healthy boundaries, seek supervision, know when to refer, and understand that there will always be something to learn. A well-trained play therapist will be able to answer "who, what, where, when, how, and why" questions regarding the treatment they provide. These answers will be greatly influenced by the identified theoretical foundation.

Table 3.1 "Who, What, When, When, and Why" of Play Therapy Treatment

	Overarching Concepts	Client/Case Specific
Who	Who am I qualified to treat? What populations will be the focus of my practice?	Who is the identified client?
What	What is the theoretical foundation which informs the mechanism of change?	What is the presenting issue/are the presenting issues? What will benefit this client to resolve/understand/learn/experience within the play therapy treatment?
Where	Where will the treatment take place? If the location varies, what are the clinical ramifications of the variability? If there are concerns, how can they be remedied?	Where will the client be seen?
When	When will treatment be provided? This includes a thoughtful examination of how many clients to see per day, how long sessions will be, how time for calls and paperwork will be scheduled, and so on.	When will treatment be provided? Are there concerns regarding missing school? Are there times which will benefit the client more (before or after visitation, etc.)?
How	How will the treatment provided follow/complement/uphold the tenets of the underlying theoretical foundation?	How will the treatment be provided? If prescriptive, how would the treatment be tailored to this particular client?
Why	Why is play therapy the treatment of choice? Why would certain interventions be more beneficial than others?	Why would the treatment proposed/provided be the best course of action for this client? Often, this is where the therapeutic powers of play would be activated.

When working to answer the "who, what, where, when, how, and why" questions regarding the provided treatment, a practitioner can address these globally as overarching concepts or per client (Table 3.1).

There are many programs, certifications, and continuing education programs available. It is important to seek out training that equates to more than a "weekend warrior" where a certificate is provided after a short period of training. Research the person or entity providing the training, look at how intensive the training is, what the requirements are, and think about what your ultimate goal is in attending. Be conscientious regarding what is needed as a clinician (knowledge, exposure, skills, etc.), what is needed personally, and what the goals are professionally. Thinking through these concepts with intention and repeating the process over time will contribute significantly to the career of the well-trained therapist.

Daniel Sweeney, PhD, RPT-S

Before talking about the key characteristics of a well-trained play therapist, I would suggest stepping back and considering the personality characteristics that are helpful for the play therapist. While fundamentally unattainable, I would endorse Landreth's (2012) suggested characteristics, which are focused on intentionality, attitudes, and motivations:

- Being *Objective and Flexible*
- Not *Judging or Evaluating*
- Being *Open-Minded*
- Being *Patient*
- Having a *High Tolerance for Ambiguity*
- Being *Future-Minded*
- Having *Personal Courage*
- Being *Real, Warmth and Caring, Acceptance, and Sensitive Understanding*
- Being *Personally Secure*
- Having a *Sense of Humor* (Landreth, 2012, pp. 99–103)

More specifically to the characteristics of a well-trained therapist, I would first defer to the requirements set forth by the Association for Play Therapy [APT] to qualify as a Registered Play Therapist [RPT] and Registered Play Therapist-Supervisor [RPT-S].

Additionally, I have some personal priorities for the training for play therapists. It has been my experience that many play therapists have what I consider to be inadequate training and knowledge in a few areas, including but not limited to the following:

- *Family systems* – It is crucial to have a systemic perspective and systemic training. This is not automatically included with all graduate mental health training programs.
- *Life span human development* – It has been my experience that there seems to be inadequate knowledge and training in life span development for many child play therapists. I would recommend consulting Ray (2016).
- *Attachment theory* – Since attachment is key in the development of both adaptive and maladaptive presentations, knowledge about these is crucial. I recommend classic and more recent literature – Bowlby and Ainsworth (Bretherton, 1992), and Mellenthin (2019).
- *Interpersonal neurobiology* – A general survey of psychoneurobiology. Some of my favorite sources include Badenoch (2008), Cozolino (2017), Kestly (2014), and Porges (2011).

- *Child/adolescent psychopharmacology* – The field of pediatric psychophar-macology is constantly and quickly evolving. Staying current in the liter-ature is crucial (Marvasti, Wu, & Merritt, 2018).
- *Parent training* – There is a wide variety of parenting approaches. Play therapists should stay current on what is available and measure its ap-propriateness and efficacy for use with parents and children. My personal preference is filial therapy (see Landreth & Bratton, 2020).

Finally, it can't be emphasized enough regarding the importance of ongoing clinical supervision in play therapy, both during and beyond the point of li-censure and certification(s).

References

Association for Play Therapy (2019). *Credentialing standards for the Registered Play Therapist: APT professional credentialing program.* https://cdn.ymaws.com/www.a4pt.org/ resource/resmgr/credentials/2020_credentials/rpt_stand_22aug2019.pdf.

Badenoch, B. (2008). *Being a brain-wise therapist: A practical guide to interpersonal neu-robiology.* W.W. Norton & Co.

Bretherton, I. (1992). The origins of attachment theory: John Bowlby and Mary Ainsworth. *Developmental Psychology, 28*(5), 759–775.

Cozolino, L. (2017). *The neuroscience of psychotherapy: Healing the social brain* (3rd ed.). W.W. Norton & Co.

Kestly, T. (2014). *The interpersonal neurobiology of play: Brain-building interventions for emotional well-being.* W.W. Norton & Co.

Landreth, G. (2002). *Play therapy: The art of the relationship* (2nd ed.). Routledge.

Landreth, G. (2012). *Play therapy: The art of the relationship* (3rd ed.). Routledge.

Landreth, G., & Bratton, S. (2020). *Child-parent relationship therapy (CPRT): An evidence-based 10-session filial therapy model* (2nd ed.). Routledge.

Marvasti, J., Wu, P. & Merritt, P. (2018). Psychopharmacology for play therapists. *International Journal of Play Therapy, 27*(1), 35–45.

Mellenthin, C. (2019). *Attachment centered play therapy.* Routledge.

O'Connor, K. J. (2016). Ecosystemic play therapy. In K. J. O'Connor, C. E. Schaefer, & L. D. Braverman (Eds.), *Handbook of play therapy* (2nd ed., pp. 195–225). Wiley & Sons.

Peabody, M. A. & Schaefer, C. E. (2016). Towards semantic clarity in play therapy. *International Journal of Play Therapy, 25*(4), 197–202.

Peabody, M. A. & Schaefer, C. E. (2019). The therapeutic powers of play: The heart and soul of play therapy. *Play Therapy, 14*(3), 4–6.

Pedersen, P. B. (1990). The multicultural perspective as a fourth force in counseling. *Journal of Mental Health Counseling, 12*, 93–95.

Porges, S. (2011). *The polyvagal theory: Neurophysiological foundations of emotions, at-tachment, communication, and self-regulation.* W.W. Norton & Co.

Ray, D. (2011). *Advanced play therapy: Essential conditions, knowledge, and skills for child practice.* Routledge.

Ray, D. (Ed.) (2016). *A therapist's guide to child development: The extraordinarily normal years.* Routledge.

Rogers, C. (1957). The necessary and sufficient conditions of therapeutic personality change. *Journal of Consulting Psychology, 21* (2), 95–103.

Schaefer, C. E. (2018, December). The 10 basic principles of prescriptive play therapy. *Play Therapy, 13*(4), 24–27.

Siegel, D. J., & Bryson, T. P. (2011). *The whole-brain child: 12 revolutionary strategies to nurture your child's developing mind.* Random House.

Sue, S. (1998). In search of cultural competence in psychotherapy and counseling. *American Psychologist, 53*(4), 440–448.

4 What Are the Top Ten Items You Feel Are Necessary in a Play Therapy Office?

Jeff Ashby, PhD, RPT-S

Ten? Is this a trick question? Seriously, it is extremely difficult (impossible?) to select only ten items/toys that are necessary to a play therapy office. There are several classic play therapy toy recommendation lists (containing more than ten items) and I would commend each of these to the reader (e.g., Axline, 1950; Landreth, 2012). They are thoughtful, well-organized, and provide thorough lists of helpful items to have in the play therapy office.

While determining the "top ten" items to have in a play therapy office is a daunting (impossible?) task, there are clear categories of items that are important to have available to the client. Kottman and Meany-Walen (2016) suggest five broad categories of items that are important to have in the playroom. These include *Scary Toys*, which offer clients the opportunity to deal with their fears; *Family/Nurturing Toys*, offering clients the chance to explore family relationships, events, and issues of nurturing; *Aggressive Toys*, that allow clients to express feelings of fear, anger, aggression, and explore issues of power and control; *Expressive Toys*, allowing clients to express creativity and symbolically work out problems and explore relationships; and *Pretend/Fantasy Toys*, which allow clients express hidden feelings, try out alternate behaviors and explore alternate roles. As all five categories of toys are important, if pressed, I would likely choose two toys from each category.

While I am, at one level, making light of the question, I do acknowledge that the selection of play therapy items for the playroom is extremely important. As Landreth (2012) notes, "Toys and materials can, however, determine or structure the kind of degree of expression by the child and their interaction with the therapist, and therefore must receive careful attention as to their selection" (pp. 138–139). Given that the items available may determine, and even limit, the degree of the child's expression, O'Connor (2005) has suggested careful consideration of whether items meet the needs of diverse play therapy clients. Whenever possible, playrooms should have culture-neutral items and culture-specific items. These might include houses that represent varying levels of socioeconomic status, figures with differing apparent ethnicities and skin hues, and varied religious symbols. If I am limited in the number of items I can have in my office (e.g., in the circumstance of needing to use a portable play kit), I would, consistent with AdPT, do my best to select items that are contextualized to the client's culture, presenting issue, and the phase of treatment.

Robert Jason Grant, EdD, RPT-S

I believe that the therapist is the most important component in the playroom and the relationship is the critical feature not a particular item. Selected toys and materials will vary depending on the population being worked with and the theoretical orientation that the play therapist is using. There are some materials I have found to be very useful with the populations (developmental disorders) I most often serve.

Playroom considerations would include constructive toys – LEGO bricks, train set, blocks, and a Mr. Potato Head. I would also have sensory toys and materials – sensory balls, weighted blanket, weighted balls, wobble and balance boards, putty, sensory tubs (sand, rice, beans, water beads), and so on. I would include functional/realistic toys – a doctor's kit, a dentist kit, a dollhouse, baby dolls, and a kitchen. In additional to these three toy categories, the following seven conceptual ideas seem important in playroom creation.

1   Varied seating options – This might include an exercise ball, small chairs, a rug, a bean bag chair. Different tactile experiences for sitting (hard, soft, bouncy, etc.)
2   Varied lighting options – The ability to change the lighting from bright to dim. Possibly using different types of lamps and shades for windows.
3   Space to move around and participate in movement-based play and interventions.
4   Adjustability – Being able to adjust and change the playroom as needed for a specific child. The ability to put away toys or have toys in open view, the ability to provide wheelchair accessibility and adjust for any disability issues.
5   Recordability and monitoring – The ability to observe through an observation window or monitoring system and the ability to record sessions as needed especially when working with parents and/or supervisees.
6   Confidentiality and privacy – Making sure that the child's play and work is confidential and cannot be heard or seen by others.
7   Client friendly – Being mindful of how the playroom might feel for a specific client coming into the playroom. How might it feel for a preschool aged child, an elementary aged child, a teen? Is the space client friendly and welcoming for the population being worked with including age, gender, and ethnicity?

Heidi Gerard Kaduson, PhD, RPT-S

While there is plenty of guidance regarding which toys to have in your playroom if you are strictly non-directive (Landreth, 2012), the prescriptive approach matches the therapy to the individual child which dictates what toys to have when needed. Therefore, for the top ten items, I would have to focus on the possibilities of generally treating children in a playroom vs. a play therapy office. When a child can come to a therapeutic playroom each week, where everything remains the same and the child's choice of play is encouraged, the child can feel truly safe. Everything in the playroom is for the child's use and with the therapeutic alliance between therapist and child, this can support the child's psychological health. Having a wider range of toys that include a hospital, a school, castles, houses, and so on can help a child gravitate toward play that allows for expression of feelings or abreactive play to slowly work through a past trauma. Although children will find a way to express themselves using whatever the therapist has, it is the existence of many of the toys that trigger the child to play out something that may be traumatic or never before spoken. I believe that when there are medical issues, it is also important to have real tools of a medical doctor – stethoscope, blood pressure cuff, needleless needles, and so on because it allows children of any age to take on the role of the doctor and play out medical issues that they may have had or will be having in the future.

One of my clients who was diagnosed on the autistic spectrum, would repeatedly play cashier, and I was instructed to shop in the playroom and bring things to him to buy. This went on for several weeks almost predictably. Then in the middle of the sixth session, he quietly went to the hospital and created a scene about a person in a hospital bed, with many tubes coming out of the body, and a large group of people, including adults and children, standing around that bed. He asked for my assistance only in finding the tubes, medicine, and so on that he needed to place in this scene. When he finished, he said, "Okay, now go shop for more toys to buy." When the session was over, I contacted the client's mom and asked her if anything seemed familiar about this scene that I described. She immediately said that it was very similar to when her mother was terminally ill in the hospital in Argentina, and this grandmother wanted all of her grandchildren to come to the hospital to see them before she died. My client was only 3 years old at the time, but his mother recalled vividly that everyone was crying, except my client. That was 7 years prior to his reenactment of that moment. He never spoke about it or showed any feelings when he was 3; however, it remained in his memory and was triggered by seeing the hospital. He played it once and was able to gain resolution. In most cases, the following would be my top ten choices of toys for a playroom:

1 Blocks
2 Expressive arts materials
3 Animal and people families (families of different ethnic groups, and animal families both wild and domestic)
4 Egg splatz balls
5 Whiteboard (with markers)
6 Baby doll with real bottle and blanket
7 Various cars and trucks (which includes rescue vehicles (police, fire, ambulance) as well as general types of cars

8   Puppets (full range to express aggression or nurturance)
9   Hospital and/or doctor's kit
10 One *Playmobil* building that could be used as home, school, hospital, and so on

Jennifer Lefebre, PsyD, RPT-S

The go-to items in my play therapy space are the sensory items – large bean bags, memory foam pillows, stuffed animals, weighted blankets, yoga mats, tubes and blankets, and a sensory basket full of "stuff" (i.e., beanbags, stress balls, putty, and slime). These items are used for regulation and grounding, and are essential for the embodied play therapy work I do, typically being used at the beginning and end of sessions by most of my clients. A variety of supplies for making slime/oobleck/playdough and other items for art (i.e., paint, markers, pastels, magazines, glue, colored paper) are also used frequently in my play therapy space, and children use them not only for expressive arts but also to self-regulate. The sand tray, a variety of miniatures, and the other items (i.e., stones, shells, nature items) that go along with it, would be a close second. These items allow for access to unconscious material in a safe, contained manner. The next items I would consider to be essential would be the play kitchen/house area (e.g., food, money, baby dolls, dress-up clothes, hats, first aid kit, medical supplies), allowing for nurturing and self-expression in order to communicate and explore relationships. Puppets would fit into this area as well. The last group of toys I feel are necessary in a play therapy room would be a doll house with corresponding human and animal families, and different types of furniture. To go along with the doll house, I have a hospital, fire station, and police station. These items are often used to demonstrate attachment and relational needs.

Clair Mellenthin, MSW, RPT-S

In my perspective, the top ten items necessary in a play therapy office outside of the traditional list of toys in play therapy literature are as follows:

1   A big, soft, comfortable pillow(s) and/or blanket. This provides for nurture and a sense of calm in the playroom. It offers a soft, comfortable place to sit on the floor to read stories in, play with various toys or make believe, and to process through challenging heartaches. This has been one of the most used "toys" over the years and used in everything from being a pirate ship cruising shark infested waters to a place where a soft, nurturing touch has been taught and implemented between a child and their parent for the first time. The blanket has been used to build a fort, wrap up a 10-year-old boy in a swaddle to be rocked by his mother, as a hideout watching out for bad guys, and as a forcefield protecting against a bloody battle and bombs raining down on us. It has also been used to snuggle up against a parent; feeling protected and simultaneously allowing for vulnerability.

2   Craft items (popsicle sticks, pom poms, chenille sticks, googly eyes, etc.) and Elmer's glue. I am a huge believer in the power of creating what you need for your play therapy work. In my playroom, these items are some of the most used outside of the traditional toys. I also bring in empty Kleenex boxes, egg cartons, toilet paper rolls, paper towel rolls, and old magazines. The process of creating what you need allows for a sense of empowerment for the child, helps to decrease the child (and parent's) defense mechanisms, and allows for access to the unconscious (Mellenthin, 2019; Perryman, Moss & Cochran, 2015).

3   Sand tray. A sand tray can be used in a variety of ways. I find that it is a very calming "toy" that can help promote self-soothing, regulation, and relaxation. When used in the traditional psychodynamic approach the sand tray and use of miniatures can be a powerful tool to access the unconscious, explore the child's personal experiences and emotions, and can increase positive parent-child interactions in play therapy.

4   A full-length child-size mirror. I have hung mine on the wall to prevent it from tipping and breaking. It is also hung so that the child can see themselves clearly and fully. I have found over the years that this has been an invaluable "toy" and used from everything from the child admiring their beautiful transformation in dress-up clothes to being used for creating a sense of self and empowerment. We have used it to practice social skills, language development, understanding and developing attunement with the parent and child, as well as being silly and playful together.

5   A feelings chart. I have a poster-size, framed (very cheap frame with a plastic cover) chart that is used on a daily basis in my playroom. I encourage play therapists to create or purchase one that uses cartoon faces instead of human faces. I use this often as part of play therapy interventions when teaching emotions, developing emotional intelligence, and promoting connection and understanding of others' emotional experiences.

6   Sensory Station. Sensory play is so important and is often overlooked in its value in the playroom. I have a shelf that contains different sensory-enhancing "toys" such as shaving cream, saline solution, bubbles, beads, dried beans, dry pasta, glue, glitter, as well as other tactile toys such as fidget toys and variety of cloth material to play with and use.

7   Wall Clock. I prefer this over a timer as it helps both the therapist and child keep track of the time. When it is always out and available, it also helps to set boundaries and limits, teach important life skills, and keeps the therapist aware and able to manage the session time appropriately.

8   Anatomically correct male and female baby dolls. These can be expensive but worth the money. Not only are they an invaluable tool in the playroom for working on sexual abuse or sexual reactivity issues, but I believe that they provide value for all children, help to decrease the stigma and shame around body parts and genitalia, as well as can be a helpful tool in teaching about nurture, family transitions and changes, as well as developing empathy and a sense of self for the child client.

9 Nerf Guns. These are allowed for playful, aggressive play that is so important for all children to experience and use to work through their own internal aggressive feelings. I also purchase the suction-tipped darts and use them in a variety of interventions – hence the need to the feelings chart to have a plastic protection (Mellenthin, 2018). I find that using these in family-based play therapy is also a very important and powerful tool to use to help work through hurts, rebuild relationships, and help the parent to become a resource and protector of their child through play.

10 Hand sanitizer and Kleenex. This helps to protect everybody from germs and illnesses, as well as can provide a nurturing experience as a child experiences an adult who cares about their well-being and will help to keep them healthy.

Akiko J. Ohnogi, PsyD

It is important to include numerous categories when choosing toys and materials for the play therapy office, such as nurturing, mending, aggressive, fantasy, creative, scary, and real life. These toys should be appropriate for various developmental age ranges, be helpful for a variety of trauma-related interventions (e.g., ships for tsunami survivors), and include items for sensory play. Based on my experience as a play therapist for over 25 years, the top ten items that I feel are necessary in a play therapy office are as follows:

1 Sofas or the equivalent. These are not necessarily to sit on but to be used when working on "safety" issues. I have had multiple children throughout the years use the two sofas I have in my office aligned in a face to face position in my play therapy room to work through their trauma experiences (e.g., surviving a natural disaster, interpersonal abuse, accidents, medical trauma, victim of kidnapping, abandonment by parents). Every single one of these children, on their own accord during unstructured play, came up with the play sequence of hopping from one sofa to the other. At times they would jump without touching the ground in between the sofas, and at other times they would try to avoid being "caught" by the play therapist while on the carpet in between. The sofas were "safe areas", while the floor in between was "dangerous". Being able to get themselves from safety point to safety point was a healing play of control over their traumatic experiences.

2 Miniatures: many clients use them for unstructured play. I also utilize them for various structured play. I do not limit the use of miniatures to sand tray work. Clients utilize these toys more often in activities other than a sand tray.

3 Playdoh (or some version of reusable clay): I utilize this medium often in structured activities and supervision.

4 Sand (kinetic): Popular with adults and children alike for use with soothing themselves through tactile and visual sensory usage.

5 Drawing materials: I utilize this more often during structured activities rather than clients choosing it of their own accord.

6 House: Popular, especially for those who are struggling with family conflict issues.

7 Large stuffed animal: Hugged often and made into "my favorite"; used as a tool to provide and receive comfort.

8 Doctor's kit: These are especially popular with clients who have experienced some form of trauma. Repeated play of gradual healing from whatever disaster, accident, illness, abuse, developmental issues, and/or interpersonal difficulties they have experienced.

9 Swords: Often used to fight off "enemies" and to feel a sense of power and control. I have various types of swords, from soft foam to huge plastic, and samurai, ninja, gladiator swords, and so on.

10 Monsters: Especially popular with clients who have experienced a trauma whether it be natural, man-made, or interpersonal. The monsters sometimes represent the disaster or perpetrator, while at other times it is the symbolization of the powerful healer/hero.

Mary Anne Peabody, EdD, RPT-S

My top ten items are materials that facilitate expression (Landreth, 2012) and include:

1 Two open wooden structures that allow the client to create a representation of a type of building (e.g., house, school, airport). I like having two to allow travel between the structures.

2 Blocks and LEGO bricks can also be used to create homes/buildings/schools or create stories in response to a directive prompt given by the therapist.

3 A box full of school materials with miniaturized versions of a chalkboard, school desks, school bus, school playground, and a variety of adult and child figures.

4 A selection of animal families to promote both nurturing/caregiving play, as well as acting out/aggressive type play.

5 Expressive props such as scarves and flowing material for role play.

6 Real life experiential toys: a medical kit; a veterinarian kit; cooking and kitchen play materials.

7 A fairly large whiteboard and chalkboard on the wall.

8 Art materials: paper, markers, crayons, model magic, and playdough.

9 A sand tray with a selection of miniatures that are easily within reach for the child.

10 I keep two or three simple board games for use in family therapy or as homework assignments after I have coached parents in emotionally responsive playing.

Dee Ray, PhD, RPT-S

For me, I need to separate the playroom from the office. Early in my play therapy career, I combined my office and playroom and found that the combination was distracting and interfered with my work in play therapy sessions, as well as my administrative work. In play therapy, I often had to set limits on office-related materials (those drawers aren't for opening, my phone is not for using, etc.) or I would be distracted by remembering an administrative task when glancing at my desk. When I concentrated on administrative work, I would be distracted by my creative juices flowing and thinking of new ways to arrange the playroom or materials that might be helpful for certain clients. Hence, I now keep my office separate from my playroom. In my office are items that help support me as a person and professional such as family photos, motivational phrases, books (lots and lots of books), small toys for me or others I supervise, and artwork. My office is about me and provides me with the self-care I need to be fully present for others.

The playroom is fully about the child. Everything in the playroom is designed to serve the needs of the child. As far as items, each toy/material is selected to provide the child a way to communicate their thoughts and feelings in a self-directed manner (Landreth, 2012). A few years back, I led a study on the most used materials in the playroom by rating the play behaviors of 68 children in play therapy who were between 3 and 10 years old (Ray et al., 2013). The top ten most used items across gender and age were (1) sandbox, (2) sand tools, (3) arts/crafts, (4) paint, (5) water, (6) kitchen, (7) puppet theater, (8) easel, (9) bop bag, and (10) hats. I found this list to correspond well to my personal preferences for items in the playroom. Most of these items allow for full expression of all feelings and themes; such as allowing children to express happiness, nurturance, power, anger, or hurt. My personal favorite is the sandbox. I believe that almost all children have some relationship with the sandbox when in play therapy. Sometimes they dive right in and use the sand to soothe themselves, sometimes they create elaborate play scenes in the sand, and sometimes they avoid the messiness and uncontrolled nature of the sand, just to name a few possibilities. The sand allows for the child to engage with a natural, organic resource to express themselves in innumerable ways.

I am also a big believer in assuring that children have access to aggressive toys or materials that allow for the expression of aggression. Children who have aggressive presenting problems necessitate materials for expression. Research has demonstrated that child-centered play therapy in which children are allowed to engage in aggressive play results in the expression of less aggression outside of the playroom (e.g., Bratton et al., 2013; Ray et al., 2009). The bop bag, aggressive animals, and weapons are essential for sending the message that children who express themselves aggressively are accepted and understood in play therapy.

Jessica Stone, PhD, RPT-S

The key concepts when discussing necessary play therapist office items are (1) therapist congruity and (2) speaking the client's language. Another important concept is that when you have included an item in the play therapy room, know it well. Play it, know it, understand it, so much so that when you are using it with a client the therapist's mind is focused on the interactions, themes, and communications, not on the mechanics of the use.

Therapist congruity is a bit more complicated than it might initially seem. This does not mean that the therapist should only include items they like. This is not the golden opportunity to create the playroom one never had as a child. Rather, congruity is a step in the fit-for-the-playroom evaluation process when considering an item for inclusion. First steps include the following: does this item tend to elicit certain interactions, information, and/or dynamics when used in play therapy? Does this item activate the therapeutic powers of play (Schaefer & Drewes, 2013)? Is this item congruent with the therapist's theoretical foundation? Does this item speak the general client's language or a specific client's language? Finally, if the item is congruent with the therapist's core belief system, it will be included in the room. If not, further self-exploration, consultation, reading, training, and/or supervision should be sought to determine if the item triggers something in the therapist which needs some attention, or if a referral might be appropriate.

The items I find to be in my top ten list are as follows (Table 4.1):

Table 4.1 Top 10 Play Therapy Items

Top 10 Play Therapy Room Items	*Examples*
1 Manipulatives	LEGO bricks
	Blocks, magnetic shapes
	Playmobil
2 Board Games	Commercial
	Professional
3 Puppets	People
	Animals
	Fantasy
	Various sizes
4 Dolls	Representative
5 Sand tray	Traditional
	Virtual
6 Digital	Tablet + apps
	Nintendo switch + games
	Virtual reality + programs
7 Dollhouse/castle/Playmobil/buildings	Various
8 Art materials	Supplies
	Paper
	Various mediums
9 Sensory	Various
10 Books	Clients
	Various topics and age ranges
	Parents/family/caregivers
	Developmental
	Diagnosis/topic specific

Daniel Sweeney, PhD, RPT-S

It is difficult – and feels impossible – for me to list the top ten items that are necessary to have in a play therapy room. Since I tend to think in categories of toys, and I like those suggested by Kottman and Meany-Walen (2016), including family/nurturing toys, scary toys, aggressive toys, expressive toys, and pretend/fantasy toys (p. 7).

Homeyer and Sweeney (2017) contend that sand tray therapy serves to create a necessary therapeutic distance for clients – that it is simply easier for a traumatized client to "speak" through one of the sand tray therapy miniature figures than to directly verbalize their pain (p. 11). They go on to assert that this therapeutic distance provides creates a safe place for abreaction to occur (p. 11). This should be true for all materials used in the play therapy process.

There is a wide variety of toys and materials that are beneficial. Though I am not limited to ten items [either in my playroom or portable tote bag of play therapy materials] – I will list ten items that I consider very important for the play therapy office. These are not listed in any order of priority.

1   Animal puppets
2   Culturally appropriate doll family
3   Animal family figures
4   Phone [at least two (real)]
5   The Lone Ranger type mask
6   Doctor's bag
7   Drum
8   Handcuffs
9   Play-Doh
10   Crayons and paper

References

Axline, V. (1950). Entering the child's world via play experiences. *Progressive Education*, *27*, 68–75.

Bratton, S., Ceballos, P., Sheely-Moore, A., Meany-Walen, K., Pronchenko, Y., & Jones, L. (2013). Head start early mental health intervention: Effects of child-centered play therapy on disruptive behaviors. *International Journal of Play Therapy, 22*, 28–42. doi:10.1037/a0030318.

Homeyer, L., & Sweeney, D. (2017). *Sandtray therapy: A practical manual* (3rd ed.). Routledge.

Kottman, T., & Meany-Walen, K. (2016). *Partners in play: An Adlerian approach to play therapy* (3rd ed.). American Counseling Association.

Landreth, G. L. (2012). *Play therapy: The art of the relationship* (3rd ed.). Routledge.

Mellenthin, C. (2018). *Play therapy: Engaging and powerful interventions for the treatment of childhood disorders.* PESI Publishing

Mellenthin, C. (2019). *Attachment centered play therapy.* Routledge

O'Connor, K. J. (2005). Addressing diversity issues in play therapy. *Professional Psychology, 36*(5), 566–573.

Perryman, K. L., Moss, R., & Cochran, K. (2015). Child-centered expressive arts and play therapy: School groups for at-risk adolescent girls. *International Journal of Play Therapy, 24*(4), 205–220.

Ray, D., Blanco, P., Sullivan, J., & Holliman, R. (2009). An exploratory study of child-centered play therapy with aggressive children. *International Journal of Play Therapy, 18*, 162–175. doi:10.1037/a0014742.

Ray, D., Lee, K., Meany-Walen, K., Carlson, S., Carnes-Holt, K., & Ware, J. (2013). Use of toys in child centered play therapy. *International Journal of Play Therapy, 22*, 43–57.

Schaefer, C. E., & Drewes, A. A. (2013). *The therapeutic powers of play: 20 core agents of change.* Wiley.

5   What Have Been Some of the Most Challenging Things You Have Experienced as a Play Therapist?

Jeff Ashby, PhD, RPT-S

I think play therapy has a lot of challenges. However, for me, the most challenging things only infrequently have to do with the actual practice of play therapy with the client. I often think of practicing play therapy as "the best of times" and "the worst of times" (Dickens, 1859/2003, p. 1). By this, I mean that nearly all times with clients are great. They're not necessarily great because things are going swimmingly. They are great because, even when things are not progressing as I would hope for the client child, it is nearly always clinically interesting. If the client is not progressing, I'm led to ask, "what am I not doing well?" or "what am I not considering?" I have the luxury and great advantage of having a network of amazing play therapists with whom I can consult. That expert consultation allows me to think actively about my conceptualization of the client, my treatment plan, my specific interventions, and my own reactions (both inside and outside of my awareness) that are impacting the work. Perhaps because I came to play therapy mid-career (or because I'm just a nerd), I am continually fascinated by nearly all aspects of the work. It is the best of times.

The practice of play therapy can also be "the worst of times". These challenging times often include the ongoing hassles of insurance, paperwork, billing issues, consents, cancellations, and no-shows. The most challenging things I've experienced as a play therapist include all of these tasks and concerns that, while important, are peripheral to the actual work of play therapy. Given the importance of parental consultation in AdPT, parents/guardians can also offer significant challenges. Issues that complicate this consultation (e.g., divorce and custody issues, reluctance to participate, triangulation with partners) can be particularly challenging for me, and it is harder for me to find these clinically interesting or enjoy the consultation process when trying to address or untangle these issues. I am particularly grateful that, for me, the actual work of play therapy (the best of times) far outweigh (and outnumber) the challenging situations (the worst of times).

Robert Jason Grant, EdD, RPT-S

I will answer this question from two perspectives, inside the playroom and outside the playroom. Inside the playroom, I have worked with many children who exhibit some extreme behaviors in play sessions. I recall a young client who came in with her parents to see me. She was diagnosed with autism, intellectual developmental disorder, and a chromosome disorder. On entering the hallway to go to the playrooms, she stopped and laid across the hallway floor and would not move for the whole session. She did this for the first five sessions. I have worked with children who crawled under chairs in the waiting room and refused to move, ran up and down the clinic hallways, busting into any closed door they could find; children running out of the clinic, children having meltdowns; and children trying to destroy the playroom. Luckily these experiences have been minimal and not the majority of what I have experienced. In each of these scenarios, the child was diagnosed with one or more developmental disorders, and the behavior was clearly diagnosis related. Nonetheless, these types of behaviors can be very challenging.

There have been many times I was not sure how to proceed or how to respond to the behavior I was seeing. In my early work as a play therapist, this would often make me uncomfortable, but through the years I have become calmer and more flexible when this type of behavior occurs. It always improves, and the most important thing I have learned is not a specific technique to address the behavior but to remain calm, not becoming stressed about any behavior and not taking the behavior personally but understanding the child is in distress, realizing the child is often dysregulated, and remembering the behavior will get better.

Outside the playroom, one of the biggest challenges has been helping people understand what play therapy is and is not. I could fill a book on the number of people and situations I have experienced who misunderstood what play therapy is and how it works. Additionally, I have experienced many professionals who say they are offering play therapy and they don't understand play therapy, have not been properly trained, and are inaccurate in what they are saying is play therapy. This has been a challenge in my local community and one I hear echoed by other play therapists across the world. It is a frustrating experience being passionate about play therapy and working hard to maintain integrity in the field and then encountering misrepresentation and inaccurate information. The best course of action I have found is to be present in my community and on social media and speak about play therapy, share information about play therapy, and work diligently to educate others about play therapy. The Association for Play Therapy provides information that is easily accessible to help educate about and promote play therapy.

Heidi Gerard Kaduson, PhD, RPT-S

I believe that one of the most difficult challenges I have had in my career as a play therapist has been concerning the parents or caregivers of my child clients. Whenever we try to help children, the playroom is the safe haven, where they work on difficulties they are having or have had in the past. However, we cannot treat children in a vacuum. Their families are of utmost importance.

Although I make it clear in my parent intake that I expect they will need to be involved, and I do not "fix" anyone, too many times the parents either lack follow-through or do not want to change anything they are doing or truly believe that it is their child that needs the work, not them. When a slow change in their child's behavior is for the better, the parent's expectations become unreasonable and too high for the child to meet, especially without their parents' help.

When it comes to the child clients, I haven't had any experiences that I would consider challenging except when a child is coming to session because they were told that therapy is so they will not behave badly in the family anymore. In this case, the child may experience play therapy as punishment. To me this means I have to make the therapy much more fun to reduce the negativity that was implanted before they began treatment. I have learned over the years that that the playfulness of the therapist can enhance the therapy to overcome this type of obstacle. I have yet to meet a child who didn't respond to the fun of play therapy. Positive emotions can enhance anyone's feelings, and that is one of the therapeutic powers that play offers.

Jennifer Lefebre, PsyD, RPT-S

Some of the most challenging things I've experienced as a play therapist have been during my experiences within the court system. My clinical practice focuses on complex developmental trauma, and most of my cases are involved in the child welfare and court systems. As such, many children I work with are in foster care or within the process of being adopted, including challenges with visitation and leading toward the termination of parental rights. As a play therapist, presenting the work I have done in the court room can often be challenging, although any type of testifying may be experienced as demanding.

The most challenging experience I have had as a play therapist was on a recent case, where the abusers were given a significantly reduced sentence initially. The children were progressing amazingly in play therapy after experiencing significant trauma. However, the abusers appealed their sentences and I found out that the court ruled in favor of the abusers because the children were "doing so well after just playing". This was heartbreaking for the adoptive family and myself. Advocating for children, and the power of play therapy, is something I am passionate about, so to see it being misrepresented or misunderstood is very challenging for me.

Clair Mellenthin, MSW, RPT-S

I think one of the most challenging experiences I have had as a play therapist is when working with parents who are in the middle of a high-conflict divorce. These parents are in an emotionally destructive pattern with one another and I find that this can supersede their ability to keep their child protected emotionally from the impact of divorce and breakup of the family unit. When a parent is in a hurt, raw place emotionally, it can be difficult to provide for the emotional needs of their child, or to understand the child's attachment needs of having a relationship with both parents (Mellenthin, 2019). In severe cases, I have experienced situations where a child has been told they have to choose what parent to live with or who they will love, as it can't be both of the parents. In other severe cases, I have had parents who have made the child change out of their clothes they wore from the other parent's home, putting these clothes in a trash bag outside until it was time for the child to return to that parent. In these cases, the parent struggled in understanding why this was detrimental to their child's mental health and well-being as they believed that they were protecting their child and loving them (more if not better than the other parent).

Other challenges I have experienced have come from the legal system, where I have been called to testify as an expert witness or due to being the child's therapist. I have experienced lawyers and judges who do not understand play therapy or believe it to be a credible form of mental health treatment. I have also had to sit for an eight hour deposition, where I was required to review every case note I had written pertaining to the children I was treating, and describe how and why I was using play therapy, what had occurred in each therapy session, and how I can make clinical assessments and judgments based on "just playing with a little kid". Early in my career, this was a much more challenging experience, as there had been little research on the efficacy of play therapy, and it was not deemed an evidence-based model of treatment. I am eternally grateful for the researchers who have dedicated themselves to this field, to be able to now have research that shows play therapy works, is empirically validated, and is an evidence-based model of mental health treatment.

Akiko J. Ohnogi, PsyD

Although there are often challenges such as trying to work with professionals who do not accept play as a therapeutic modality or even those who "do not believe" in psychotherapy, the most challenging things I have experienced as a play therapist have by far been related to cases – typically when parents are battling over their child. In particular, I have had to deal with much stress due to cases where some form of child custody issue has been present. Due to this, I specify on my website and I am upfront with parents that I will not write reports for court and I will only provide psychological treatment with this understanding.

I have had quite a few requests for reports from parents who are referred to me by attorneys. In the past I would only write general information about the effects that acrimonious divorces have on children. I would specify particular information based on the gender and age of the child(ren). At this point I will no longer write any type of report. It takes away time from being able to treat the children on my caseload.

My decision to forgo any cases that involve report writing for courts is due to having had cases where families would come in stating a desire for treatment for their child effected by an acrimonious divorce, yet ultimately the parents were relying on my reports to win their court case. Numerous parents became so reliant on these reports for court that they would only bring in their children so that I would have updated information on how they are doing and therefore request I write more reports for the court. Parents of current clients sign a treatment agreement which indicates they will neither ask for reports for court nor subpoena me to testify on behalf of anyone.

Mary Anne Peabody, EdD, RPT-S

I have provided play therapy in a number of settings including children's hospitals, public elementary school settings, nonprofit agencies, and private practice. By far the most demanding, yet the most important setting in my opinion has been the school setting. Due to many children not being able to access community-based therapists, and if they receive any services at all, it will most likely occur in the school setting (Brueck, 2016). There are challenges and barriers to implementing play therapy in schools, as well as strategies to overcome these barriers (Ray, 2010). When I practiced in schools, there was a macro-level devaluing of play in general and standardized testing was privileged over playful pedagogical approaches. Fortunately, the pendulum is now shifting as school personnel are realizing the importance of social and emotional learning (Durlak et al., 2015) trauma-informed practices (Thomas et al., 2019) and play-based learning (Lynch, 2015).

Another challenge as a play-based consultant for schools nationally and internationally was the realization that while society likes to talk about preventative mental health in children, rarely does funding follow. There appears to be a "treatment over prevention mentality" when resources are scarce. I understand that children with externalizing behaviors need help for their safety and the safety of others, and that not all social and emotional issues are preventable. Yet, I remain a prevention advocate and believe in addressing some issues early by bringing a systematic focus on the early identification and treatment of the youngest of children through play-based interventions (Peabody et al., 2018). We should simply work harder to prioritize prevention efforts before they become crystallized and more difficult to treat. The establishment of a registered school-based play therapy credential is an important first step in what needs to be an on-going movement to address the play therapy service delivery gap of both prevention and treatment services in our elementary schools.

Dee Ray, PhD, RPT-S

I have experienced challenging children, parents, and settings over my time as a play therapist. Of course, there are times in which I struggled with certain behaviors but mostly I find those types of challenges to be inspirational and motivating for my work. My most considerable challenges have more to do with my personal and internal conflicts related to working with the vulnerable population of children. I was attracted to the field of child therapy as an advocate for children, wanting to support individual children while changing the world to be more effectively responsive to children. Although I have learned healthy boundaries over the years and value children's innate abilities to move toward self- and other-enhancing ways-of-being, I am still internally conflicted with the need to rescue or save children. When I see the needs of my clients go unmet, denied, or rejected, I experience a twinge of overresponsibility that I need to be the one to save this child. Early in my career, this need to rescue was detrimental to my work-life balance as I would become preoccupied with what was happening with my child clients and what I needed to be doing to help, often feeling distressed in my inability to save them.

Through time and experience, I learned that my role is not savior or hero, but my role is to journey with children as they navigate their circumstances and environments because I have seen that they are capable of working through adverse conditions. Yet, even in late career, I still struggle with the little voice inside my head that says I need to change the world for children and I should be doing this all the time. I deal with this little voice through writing, presenting, and teaching in hopes that these activities are appropriate outlets for making a difference on a larger scale.

Jessica Stone, PhD, RPT-S

After some thought, the list of challenging things I have experienced as a play therapist is longer than I initially expected. Play therapy has some unique outside-the-playroom and within-the-playroom challenges due to the common misconceptions regarding the work. Overarching, I believe there are two distinct arenas of these external challenges:

1 various populations not understanding how play can be healing when key tenets of play therapy are applied to the therapeutic process (other professionals in the community, insurance companies, etc.) and
2 a wide range of variability in the quality and scope of training regarding play therapy which results in play therapy having different meanings and presentation in any given arena (for instance, I taught very briefly for a training site which had only presented one theory of play therapy and the students at the end of their six-course program were not even aware that there were other theories of play therapy. Whatever a therapist's theoretical foundation, it is very important to be well versed in the fundamentals of many play therapy theories).

Within the treatment process, play therapists can experience challenges when working with the various systems which effect the client (caregivers, school, other providers, governmental bodies, etc.). There are portions of these dynamics which are the responsibility of the play therapist and therefore within their control, and other portions which are not. For example, a play therapist can attempt to work with caregivers from numerous angles, request meetings, provide guidance and resources but often has no control regarding the appropriate follow-through by the caregiver. Another example would be a play therapist who did not front-load the theoretical underpinnings of the work with the family so there is a lack of understanding regarding the power of play, the process of play therapy, and the therapeutic goals.

Daniel Sweeney, PhD, RPT-S

Although I am not as experienced as many of my colleagues, I have been doing play therapy for some 32 years. I have actually had very few challenging things occur *inside* of the play therapy room. While I have had challenging clients, I have great confidence in play therapy as a modality and great confidence in the *process* of play therapy. This is obviously not to say that I have had nothing but success with all of my play therapy clients. This has not been, nor ever will be, my experience as a therapist. I have had to refer clients that have required greater or more specific expertise, have had premature terminations, and have not seen as much progress as I would have preferred. I have, however, not seen these as challenges.

Where I have experienced challenges as a play therapist is not so much with child clients but with their parents. I have encountered more resistance and noncompliance with parents than I have with children. I would often like to use a parenting intervention, such as filial therapy, and have too often encountered reticence, resistance, or refusal. Some parents are simply too focused on an expert "fixing" their "damaged" child and not willing to explore the etiology of the presenting issue. Having said this, I recognize that many parents are exhausted and dealing with their own challenges beyond their children's problems.

Another "challenging thing" comes to mind when I ponder my play therapy career is something that moves outside of the realm of therapy. When there was an intersection of the ages of my own children with the ages of my child clients, I experienced feelings of transference I had not prepared for. When I was working with severely traumatized and abused children – and came home to be with my own children of the same ages – I experienced tugs on my emotions that I was not expecting. I felt an increased need to hold and protect my own children, sometimes tearing up at home as I recognized the safety enjoyed by my own children but not available to my child clients. This occurred primarily when I was working with severely traumatized children in therapeutic foster children. To a lesser degree, I feel some of that today, as I have young grandchildren. Since I am only a part-time practitioner, however, this feeling is somewhat rare.

References

Brueck, M. K. (2016). Promoting access to school-based services for children's mental health. *American Medical Association Journal of Ethics, 18*(12), 1218–1224.

Dickens, C. (1859/2003). *A tale of two cities.* Penguin Books.

Durlak, J. A., Domitrovich, C. E., Weissberg, R. P., & Gullotta, T. P. (2015). *Handbook of social and emotional learning: Research and practice.* Guilford Publishing.

Lynch, M. (2015). More play please: The perspective of kindergarten teachers on play in the classroom. *American Journal of Play, 7*(3), 347–370.

Mellenthin, C. (2019). *Attachment centered play therapy.* Routledge

Peabody, M. A., Perryman, K., Hannah, M., Smith, L., & Sanyshyn, S. (2018) Improving mental health outcomes for young children through the implementation of primary project. *Journal of School-based Counseling Policy and Evaluation, 1*(1) 40–50.

Ray, D. (2010). Challenges and barriers to implementing play therapy in schools. In A. A. Drewes and C. E. Schaefer (Eds.), *School-based play therapy* (2nd ed., pp. 87–104). Wiley & Sons.

Thomas, S. M., Crosby, S., & Vanderhaar, J. (2019). Trauma-informed practices in schools across two decades: An interdisciplinary review of research. *Review of Research in Education, 43,* 422–452.

6 What Are Your Thoughts about Using Technology in Play Therapy?

Jeff Ashby, PhD, RPT-S

As noted in a variety of places (e.g., Stauffer, 2018), technology's place in play therapy is somewhat controversial. When I consider the use of technology in play therapy, I am moved to ask, "how can you keep it out of the playroom?" That is, technology use among children is ubiquitous (American Academy of Pediatrics, 2016). One example of this is that I used to try to be aware of popular children's cartoons so that I could understand references children made or characters or plot lines they were reproducing in art or imaginative play, I am now compelled to try and keep up the most popular video games (e.g., Kottman et al., 2018). My awareness of the prominent characters and plot lines in video games and other social media can help me in the first phase of AdPT, building the relationship, as it can be a place of common ground and meeting clients where they are. Understanding the language of technology (and especially video games) also helps me in the second phase of AdPT, understanding the child's lifestyle. If I can quickly grasp the terminology the client is using or identify the characters or plot lines that the child is depicting in a variety of media (e.g., art or sand), I'm more quickly able to understand how the child may be relating to the characters and plot lines. This understanding can also help me in developing metaphors and speaking the client's language in the third and fourth phases of AdPT, helping the clients gain understanding into their lifestyle and reorientation/reeducation.

I am open to using technology in play therapy interventions. As an Adlerian play therapist, I use a combination of nondirective and directive interventions. In large part due to its strong draw for some clients, I do not have technology available for the client to choose in times of unstructured play. However, just as I might bring a specific book or game to a session, I may selectively use technology in the third or fourth phases of AdPT to develop insight, build a skill, practice a new behavior, or develop a metaphor. Kottman (cited in Stauffer, 2018) notes that "specific video games can be used to provide a way to … practice targeted skills (like cooperation, anxiety management, and frustration tolerance strategies) that can be applied to other outside-the-playroom situations and relationships" (p. 23). I have the same criteria for choosing technology for use in the playroom that I would have for traditional games (e.g.,

Jenga, pick-up sticks) or any other cooperative technique. The choice of intervention is intentional and, unlike most other techniques, I often let parents/guardians know that I am using the technology because I want to anticipate any concerns they might have ("We are paying you to play video games with our child?").

Robert Jason Grant, EdD, RPT-S

I use different forms of technology in my play therapy work. Mostly I implement technology-based play with the children and adolescents I work with who have been diagnosed with ASD and other developmental disorders. Research focused on ASD and technology interventions has provided several positive findings. Currently, there is an ever increasing, rapid emergence of new technologies, especially those created as interventions for ASD (Grant, 2019).

When I am considering a technology-based intervention or type of play for children and adolescents with ASD, I am recognizing the natural draw toward technology for many on the spectrum and recognizing the creative possibilities to utilize technology in the therapy process. Research results have provided evidence for the overall effectiveness of technology-based interventions, support for continuing development, evaluation, and clinical usage of technology-based interventions with the ASD population (Grynszpan, Weiss, Perez-Diaz, & Eynat, 2013).

For example, an adolescent whom I worked with was diagnosed with ASD. He was considered more severe in terms of his skill deficits and functioning ability. He was having challenges with becoming dysregulated and angry and when he would get in this state, he would often become physical with his parents. This was becoming a very problematic situation as he could hurt himself or his parents. We began working on regulation strategies with many interventions not being successful. He had an iPad that he often used, and I decided to try and use a deep breathing app (Breath2Relax). I downloaded the app on his iPad and showed him the app. We practiced the app together and he was very responsive. He seemed to be more interested than usual, likely because we were using his iPad. I also explained the app to his parents and instructed them to support him using his app at home when he needed to relax or calm. We would practice using the app at the beginning and end of each session and he began using it on his own at home. The breathing app actually became his primary coping skill that he would use to help him regulate. His dysregulated and anger behavior greatly reduced once he began using the breathing app. I was able to introduce other sensory and regulation apps to him and we began improving his ability to recognize and express emotions through this type of tablet play.

Although there is quite a bit of research related to using technology with children and adolescents with ASD, we need more research in using technology in play therapy across issues and diagnosis and especially in conjunction with our seminal play therapy theories. Technology use in therapy would have to be a personal decision. If a therapist were not comfortable with technology, then it would not be a good fit. It also doesn't have to look one way. Play therapists should work within their own comfort level and knowledge base. They should feel empowered to explore the use of technology in the playroom and feel equally satisfied deciding to bypass technology play.

Heidi Gerard Kaduson, PhD, RPT-S

I am a believer in using whatever works, and technology is the new way children talk through their play. Therefore, I believe it is another tool to use with certain types of children including but not limited to children with attention-deficit hyperactivity disorder (ADHD) or executive functioning difficulties, children with sensory integration disorder, as well as children with dyslexia. Technology has much to offer children and their interest in it allows for treatment to be used through the technology of choice. As play therapists, we should be able to use the metaphor in any game or app to help a child heal. They certainly learn skills for executive functioning easily through many of the games they enjoy playing (i.e., Minecraft).

Children can learn self-regulation by playing any of the games technology has to offer. In my practice, I have had several children work on emotional regulation while losing a game. Over time, we can play together, and I model the self-talk and deep breathing so they can work through the impulses they used to have such as throwing the controller when they were losing or angry. When a child needs to do sand tray work, and it is clear they want to, but they cannot tolerate the sand, I use the Virtual Sandtray App (VSA) (Stone, 2016). I have tried different types of sand, but the VSA has much to offer the child, including any type of character, place, or thing and all situations that the child wants to play out are easily accessible. I have seen children gravitate to the VSA when they know it exists, and they feel they can master it easily without having the sensory disruption of touching the sand or spraying the sand, both of which disturbs them. Children with learning disabilities often feel competent with technology, which is contrary to the way they feel in school settings. They can teach me how to play a game, and reinforce for themselves the knowledge they have, the planning they do, and the success of winning the game.

Jennifer Lefebre, PsyD, RPT-S

Technology is not within my comfort zone, as I am not very tech-savvy. I often joke about this with my adolescent clients, and they seem to enjoy teaching me about technology, which builds their competencies and feelings of self-worth. Using technology as a way to connect with my adolescent clients, in order to see and experience what is important in their world, has been my favorite way to include technology. Several of my clients will pull up their social media accounts or photos to show me pieces of their world, which was never a possibility before technology.

I use music often in therapy and have created playlists with my clients. We think about if the music "hypes or calms" them (i.e., is it up-or-down regulating), and will change the icon or attach a picture to help them access the song when needed. At times, we will tag their friends or family members in the list, and attach their contact, so that if the client needs to quickly access a support person or friend they can.

Although I prefer hands-on collages, the creation of virtual vision boards has been a fun process with my clients. Additionally, I have utilized characters of interest in the play therapy room from video games to incorporate technology. I have made game cards with clients that show coping skills, strengths, and challenges for them and their family and friends – creating a game where we can play out social situations and relationships. These cards are based on the skills sets of the video games in which my clients have interest.

I would like to get more comfortable with the use of technology in the play therapy room, as I can see its value in many arenas, and I know this is an area of growth in our field. One of the ways I am doing this is by expanding my own use of technology in my personal life. I am getting more comfortable using electronics in general, and I am learning about gaming from my children and their friends. I am creating memes for the expression of emotions with an adolescent client on with pictures he has taken. I am hoping to learn more from some of my clients, as it helps to build their competency to teach me also!

Clair Mellenthin, MSW, RPT-S

I think there is a place and time for the use of technology in play therapy and I tend to take the child's lead in the introduction or allowance for it in the play therapy process. I find that for many older children, tweens, and teens, this is an especially important aspect of their world and while some may need a break from it during sessions, for others, this can be a critical component to their treatment and progress. If it is important to the child, it is important to me. I find that I need to be up to date on what is popular and the "cool" thing for the moment with regards to YouTube videos, video games and apps, as this helps me to relate and converse with some of the kids on my caseloads. Others want nothing to do with it and are happy to use and engage in traditional play therapy methods and process.

I do tend to use a lot of media and technology in my play therapy practice with tweens and teens. We will watch YouTube videos in session to look up lyrics to songs, find music or videos that help the client identify different thoughts and feelings, as well as make sense of their experiences both socially and emotionally. I have used different YouTube videos and shorts in group therapy, individual therapy, and family therapy where we will watch the video together, process the content, explore different thoughts and feelings, and then use this as a foundation for creating expressive arts or for group interventions. There are also some fabulous videos for guided imagery, regulation, and self-soothing that both I and my clients enjoy bringing into the therapy sessions.

With younger children, I find that those who want to use technology in the play therapy process also are trying to show me what is important to them and in their world. In play therapy, there have been many times over the years that Minecraft has become an important tool. The children (young and old) enjoy teaching me how to play, and most importantly, have loved showing me the worlds they have created. In this sense, we are creating Lowenfeld's World Technique (1979) utilizing technology instead of sand and miniatures. We identify the strengths, challenges, hurts, and joys the child experiences as well as can use the different parts of the game as metaphor and symbolism. For example, in Minecraft Survival Mode, there is a Creeper which can show up unexpectedly and ruin what you have created or kill your character. For many kids, we have used this as a metaphor for the unexpected and/or ongoing challenges they face in their real life and create coping strategies to use when they encounter "their Creeper". This has been a fun, playful way to teach healthy anger management and affect regulation strategies, work through trauma, and increase self-awareness with children.

Akiko J. Ohnogi, PsyD

I believe that if used properly, technology can be a strong tool especially with the exposure and emphasis on technology in our cultures. It is important that technology not be used if the play therapist is not comfortable with it, and/or does not know how to use it effectively.

I do take workshops at conferences from time to time to keep myself updated on how others are utilizing technology in their treatment. I am not an active technology user (in my professional or personal life). At most, I use technological tools to email, Skype with clients, consult with other professionals, and for clinical supervision. I do encourage supervisees and trainees to look into the possibilities of utilizing technology. Although I cannot teach them myself, I will incorporate video game storylines into other forms of play and activities (creating a scene out of clay, role-playing, etc.) even though I am not using the video game itself within sessions.

Occasionally, teenagers play music on their smartphone so that I know what music they like. Other than smartphones for sharing music, I have not had anyone bring their technology equipment into the play therapy room (except to take photographs of their creations or to show me messages between themselves and someone they are telling me about). If they wanted to "show me" a video game, I would allow it if we could use it therapeutically (e.g., work on friendship issues, family conflict, self-esteem, emotional outbursts). I do not provide technology on my own or suggest it for my clients.

Mary Anne Peabody, EdD, RPT-S

I am open to the concept that digital play therapy is simply another tool (Stone & Ehrig, 2019). As the play landscape for children continues to change, children appear to have less exposure to and familiarity with expressive toys from previous generations (Brown & Vaughn, 2009). If technology is offered as "just another tool" in the selection of playroom materials, I believe children will choose it because of its familiarity in what is initially an unfamiliar environment. Finding something familiar to engage with early in the play therapy process offers a sense of safety which precedes relationship building. While our play materials and toys are the tools that invite children to enter the play therapy relational process, it is the combination of the therapists' presence, responsiveness, and the powers of play that drive the desired change. Given this belief, it should not matter what play medium or tool is used as long as you can help build a therapeutic alliance to initiate, facilitate, or strengthen change.

Digital technologies have already changed our way of life, ways of communication, channels of influence on others, and social behavior. It is embedded in all we do, and the possibilities are certainly promising. I plan to continue to grow professionally in my knowledge and use of technology within the many therapeutic spaces we encounter. I remain especially intrigued about the use of technology in children's hospitals where play opportunities can often be limited and think this context is especially fertile ground for digital play therapy research (Bakker, Janssen & Noordam, 2018).

Another place for extending technology usage is in the realm of supervision. I was very fortunate to receive advanced training in "supervision of play therapy supervision" where technology was used to polish my supervisory skills. Advances in technology has made the digital recording of our work so easy. The ability to deconstruct your own gestures, word choice, missed opportunities, and important therapeutic supervisory turning points remains one of the greatest learning opportunities that technology offers us. The digital advances also have allowed supervisors the ability to offer distance supervision enabling connections across geographic locations. The possibilities for technology use in play therapy have only just begun.

Dee Ray, PhD, RPT-S

My thoughts on using technology in the play room are decidedly negative. As a child-centered play therapist, I believe that the relationship between the therapist and child is the healing agent of change. Each material in the playroom is selected to support this relationship, a dynamic back-and-forth interaction between the child and therapist in real life. Although I understand that technology, video games, and so on may be used to teach children certain skills, I do not see my role as teacher but as a facilitator of relationship. There are many places in which children are taught knowledge and skills by an adult but that is not my role as I see it. My role is to provide an environment in which a child feels heard and understood, cared about and trusted. This relationship requires full presence from both the therapist and child. The use of video gaming in play sessions may allow a therapist and child to interact, but it is void of therapeutic contact, the type of contact in which I, as the play therapist, make myself fully available to the child with warmth, acceptance of the child, and authenticity, to psychologically, emotionally, or spiritually touch and be touched (Schmid, 2002) in order to open an environment for the child to engage in an interpersonal process.

In addition to my perspective that technology is likely to interfere with the therapeutic relationship I seek to build, I also consider the American Academy of Pediatrics recommendation that children should spend two or less hours per day in sedentary screen time due to links between screen usage and obesity, sleep disruption, negative academic effects, and decrease in desire for real-life relationships (Council on Communications and Media, 2016). However, children typically spend over three hours a day engaged with a screen (Chen & Adler, 2019). I do not believe that play therapy should be another place that children are encouraged to overuse screen time and avoid the joys and complications of real-life relationships. Outside of the playroom, I attempt to stay current with the latest video games, apps, social media, and television shows that appeal to children in order to provide better understanding of the child when they talk about or show me (in the waiting room) their interests. I also stay current with technology in order to provide parent consultation regarding the struggles parents endure as they navigate raising their tech-savvy children in a high technology world.

Jessica Stone, PhD, RPT-S

On a fundamental level I believe the focus of speaking our client's language, entering their world, honoring their culture, and abiding by our ethical bounds to create a safe and accepting environment by definition requires play therapists to responsibly include technology in play therapy. If a client presents for therapeutic mental health treatment and the practitioner rejects part of their culture, part of who they are, what they are interested in, the language they "speak" – then they are essentially rejecting a portion of *who the client is*. If the client feels rejection, then I strongly question whether or not the therapy will be the open, accepting, honoring, nurturing, safe experience play therapists are seeking.

Frequently, the concerns regarding the use of technology in play therapy are more about the therapist's discomfort, lack of knowledge, and lack of experience. There is also much conversation about the confusing research as of 2020 regarding the pros and cons of technology use in general. The research is difficult to wade through for certain. Unfortunately, much of the research to date is poorly executed, poorly defined, and reported with enormous confirmation bias. Hopefully the years to come will provide much more well-constructed research with little to no confirmation bias involved. Amy Orben and Andrew

Pryzybylski of the Oxford Internet Institute have been diligently working through enormous literature searches to identify quality research in these areas (University of Oxford for the Oxford Internet Institute, 2016).

Several authors have written about the therapeutic benefits of incorporating technology and gaming in therapy and the importance of well-done research (Bean, 2018; Ferguson, 2015; Kowert & Quandt, 2016; Madigan, 2016; Stone, 2019a, 2020). Character choice and development, meaningful game play, themes, story lines, social dynamics, team skills, and more are extremely powerful within a variety of games and applications. The therapeutic processes and information offers invaluable windows into important psychological arenas.

The pros and cons of technology's place in society, the importance of balance in all our lives, and the effects of such technology on our bodies and minds are all critical concepts. However, this should not be the basis for inclusion or exclusion in the play therapy setting. For now, and in the foreseeable future, technology is here to stay. The use of and integration in our day to day lives for business, entertainment, and learning in increasing exponentially. The important focus now is how do we appropriately incorporate these tools into play therapy, not whether or not the use of technology is good for humankind – and therefore our clients – when discussing in session use (parental consultation regarding familial usage and balance is a different topic and dependent on the family's values and needs).

For people with interest in these areas, the inclusion of technological tools allows for the use of highly motivating mediums which equates to high engagement. These are incredibly powerful ways for play therapists to understand what the client's world is like, how they see themselves in the world, what their place is, boundaries, identity, and so much more. The inclusion of properly vetted, therapeutically appropriate digital tools in play therapy by a clinician who understands the program(s) well and can identify the therapeutic powers of play activated, will greatly enhance the play therapy relationship and progress. Digital tools have a very powerful place in play therapy.

Daniel Sweeney, PhD, RPT-S

While I do not currently use technology in play therapy, I have no objections whatsoever to using it when developmentally appropriate – with older children and adolescents. I do remain somewhat reticent about its use with young children. I have many colleagues who have used technology quite effectively in the play therapy process. I would refer the reader to Jessica Stone's (2019b) book *Integrating Technology into Modern Therapies*.

I had the opportunity to write the Foreword to Stone's (2019b) book and asserted that

> If therapy is based on relationship, and the basic relational tool is empathy – which is entering into the client's world – is it possible that technology can practically facilitate and perhaps enhance this "entering"

process? Psychotherapists use a variety of tools to facilitate the entering process – why shouldn't technology be one of these tools? Since technology has long been [and will continue to be] a pervasive part of the world we live in, should it really be avoided in the mental health process? The simple answer is: of course not!

(Sweeney, 2019, p. xii)

Additionally, I agree with Hull's (2015) proposed benefits for the use of technology in the therapeutic process, including (1) making the therapy room more inviting and the process of therapy less threatening; (2) providing a foundation for bonding between therapists and clients; (3) building opportunities for the use of imagination and creativity; (4) offering opportunities for therapeutic metaphors and life applications; and (5) allowing for a greater understanding of the client's strengths and weaknesses, along with a platform on which these can be improved (pp. 616–617).

I look forward to my own further exploration to the use of technology in the play therapy process. I also encourage readers to become adequately trained and supervised in this process before using technology with children. There is great potential.

References

American Academy of Pediatrics (2016). Policy statement: Media and young minds. *Pediatrics, 138*(5), e1–e5. http://pediatrics.aappublications.org/content/pediatrics/138/5/e20162591.full.pdf.

Bakker, A., Janssen, L., & Noordam, C. (2018). Home to hospital live streaming with virtual reality goggles: A qualitative study exploring the experiences of hospitalized children. *Journal of Medical Internet Research: JMIR Pediatrics and Parenting, 1*(2), e10. https://doi:10.2196/pediatrics.9576.

Bean, A. M. (2018). *Working with video gamers and games in therapy: A clinician's guide.* Routledge.

Brown, S. & Vaughn, C. (2009). *Play: How it shapes the brain, opens the imagination, and invigorates the soul.* Penguin Group.

Chen, W., & Adler, J. (2019). Assessment of screen exposure in young children, 1997 to 2014. *JAMA Pediatrics, 173*(4), 391–393. doi:10.1001/jamapediatrics.2018.5546.

Council on Communications and Media (2016). Media use in school-aged children and adolescents. *Pediatrics, 138*(5), e20162592. https://doi.org/10.1542/peds.2016-2592.

Ferguson, C. J. (2015). Do Angry Birds make for angry children? A meta-analysis of video game influences on children's mental health, prosocial behavior, and academic performance. *Perspectives on Psychological Science, 10*(5), 646–666.

Grant, R. J. (2019). Utilizing technology interventions with children and adolescents with autism spectrum disorder (ASD). In J. Stone (Ed.), *Integrating technology into modern therapies: A clinician's guide to developments and interventions* (pp. 124–136). Routledge.

Grynszpan, O., Weiss, P. L., Perez-Diaz, F., & Eynat, G. (2013). Innovative technology-based interventions for autism spectrum disorder: A meta-analysis. *Autism, 18*(4), 346–361.

Hull, K. (2015). Technology in the playroom. In K. O'Conner, C. Schaefer, & L. Braverman (Eds.), *Handbook of play therapy* (2nd ed., pp. 613–627). Wiley.

Kottman, T., Petersen, N., Kottman, J., & Lavenz, B. (2018). *How to talk so gamers will listen and listen so gamers will talk: Using the language of vice games in play therapy and counseling*. The Encouragement Zone.

Kowert, R., & Quandt, T. (2016). *The video game debate*. Routledge.

Lowenfeld, M. (1979). *Understanding children's sandplay: Lowenfeld's world technique*. Allen and Unwin.

Madigan, J. (2016). *Getting gamers: The psychology of video games and their impact on the people who play them*. Rowman & Littlefield.

Schmid, P. (2002). Presence: Im-media-te co-experiencing and co-responding. Phenomenological dialogical and ethical perspectives on contact and perception on person-centred therapy and beyond. In G. Wyatt & P. Sanders (Eds.), *Rogers' therapeutic conditions: Evolution, theory and practice Volume 4: Contact and perception* (pp. 182–203). PCCS.

Stauffer, S. D. (2018). Technology in play therapy: A collegial debate between seven veteran play therapists. *Play Therapy*, September, 20–23.

Stone, J. (2016). *Virtual Sandtray App*. https://www.sandtrayplay.com/Press/Virtual-SandtrayArticle01.pdf.

Stone, J. (2019a). Digital games. In J. Stone & C. E. Schaefer (Eds.), *Game play* (3rd ed.). Wiley.

Stone, J. (Ed.). (2019b). *Integrating technology into modern therapies*. Routledge.

Stone, J. (2020). *Digital play therapy: A clinician's guide to comfort and competence*. Routledge.

Stone, J. & Ehrig, M. (2019). *Just another tool: Digital Play Therapy*. Workshop presentation at the International Play Therapy Study Group, Wroxton, England.

Sweeney, D. (2019). Foreword. In J. Stone (Ed.), *Integrating technology into modern therapies* (pp. xi–xiii). Routledge.

University of Oxford for the Oxford Internet Institute (2016). *Research*. https://www.oii.ox.ac.uk/research/.

Part II

Process

S

7 What Emphasis Do You Place on the Importance of Speaking the Client's Language?

Jeff Ashby, PhD, RPT-S

I would argue that speaking the client's language is of utmost importance because, as Landreth (2012) notes, play is the language used in play therapy. For me, this has been consistently illustrated in doing group play therapy, with adventure therapy techniques with newly arrived refugee children (Ashby et al., 2008). Despite the absence of a shared verbal language (as newly arrived refugees, most clients had very limited English skills, which is my only language), we were able to communicate through play. While some processing of adventure techniques took place through translators, much of the actual communication took place through play.

One of the important things that clients communicate through their play is their preferences with regard to toys or play therapy media. For instance, I learn quickly whether clients are drawn to the sand tray, to puppets, to art supplies, and/or to more active games or play. As I am formulating more directive interventions to help the client gain insight (phase three of AdPT) or facilitate reorientation/reeducation (phase four of AdPT), I will often use the toys/medium to which the clients seem most drawn. For instance, with a client who seems drawn to puppets during nondirected play, I might engage in storytelling with puppets (as in the case of Creative Characters, Brooks, 1981).

Learning to speak the language of the client is also important to me because of the high value I place on metaphor. Clients are consistently communicating through metaphors. This "symbolic language" (Mills & Crowley, 2014) gives clients an indirect way to communicate their thoughts, feelings, attitudes, and experiences (Kottman & Ashby, 2002). It is important to me to understand, and in many cases use the language of, the client's metaphors. Speaking the client's metaphorical language, often communicated through role plays, stories, puppet shows, sand trays, and artwork, helps me build a relationship with the client and gain insight into the client's lifestyle. I can also use that metaphorical language to design interventions for helping the client gain insight and reorientation/reeducation.

An important intervention in AdPT is metacommunication about patterns or themes in the clients' lives connected to clients' conceptualization

(Kottman & Meany-Walen, 2016). In metacommunication, the play therapist makes interpretive guesses about the child's strengths or assets, family dynamics, relationship patterns, problem-solving strategies, and other aspects of the child's lifestyle that might be out of the child's awareness and/or might be getting in the way of optimal functioning. Metacommunication is a "hallmark skill" of AdPT (Kottman, personal communication November 25, 2019) that requires the play therapist to have insight into the client's lifestyle. This insight is primarily garnered from the child's communication through play. As a result, speaking the client's language, is extremely important to my work in play therapy.

Robert Jason Grant, EdD, RPT-S

Speaking the child's language involves understanding that children "speak" through play. This is one of the essential features, understandings, and implementations of any play therapy theory or approach. Landreth (1991) stated that anyone who has ever been in the presence of children for any extended period of time is well acquainted with the personality and behavioral variability they exhibit as they go about exploring their world in their own individual, unique ways. Much of this exploration is done through play which can take on many manifestations.

I believe that speaking the client's language, specifically when the client is a child, means understanding a child will play in ways that mean something to them and this play is important and should be allowed. For the therapist, the goal is to value the play and not limit it, not control it, or extinguish it. This is not always easy. Some therapists may be uncomfortable with certain types or preferences of play a child may gravitate toward. There may also be a temptation to manipulate the play to lead the child where the therapist feels he or she needs to go. There may also be outside pressures for the therapist to correct or "fix" an issue and produce results within a certain number of sessions, all of which could hinder the child's natural play exploration.

The play therapist has a responsibility to allow the child's language of play to manifest, understanding the manifestation of play in children is widely defined and realized. Many children will present with purposeful symbolic and pretend play, but I have also worked with children who gravitated toward functional play with another person. They want and seem to need another person to play with them. Other children need help learning how to play; their desire is present, but they do not fully understand how to "speak their language" and they need to be taught. Others want to play in very specific ways such as with board games, or expressive arts approaches, or movement play. The play language can also look differently with regard to the age of the child, culture, and developmental level.

Speaking the client's language is ultimately about acceptance, that is, joining into the child's world without judgment, whether that be accepting a certain type of play, accepting that the child does not play and allowing literal verbal communication, being less directive, or being more directive. It's about allowing the child to be in their world and being willing to adapt and be what the child needs us to be as they speak their language of play.

Heidi Gerard Kaduson, PhD, RPT-S

Play is the only language that children naturally use to process their difficulties. It is universal, so there is no need to speak their primary verbal language. However, the culture of the child must be known and understood before starting to use play therapy with them. Different cultures have unique traditions and types of play that the therapist must know of before beginning the play therapy treatment. Even the most verbal child may not be able to access their own feelings about difficulties in their lives. Certainly, when a child is in the preoperational stage of cognitive development, their verbal ability may be very high, but they are not socially or emotionally at the same level. I make sure to ask most children who are very verbal what they mean after they say a phrase that seems unusually mature. In almost all cases, they do not know what it meant (usually illustrated with, "I don't know"). In contrast to "talking" with a child, it is much more important for the play therapist to be playful. Playfulness may be silent, nonverbal, or verbal but involves conveying enthusiasm and motivation for, and with, the child; a willingness to engage with the child and their ideas in whatever manner the child desires; and providing them with the freedom to choose and try out new ideas (McInnes, 2019). By listening to and observing children's views of play, it enables the play therapist to understand the language of the child and thereby follow that child's play to allow for the healing to continue through the child's own language, which is play.

Jennifer Lefebre, PsyD, RPT-S

I feel it is an honor as a play therapist to be invited into the lives of the families we work with, so using their language is of the upmost importance to me. This goes beyond the understanding that we view the toys as the words of the child and play as their language (Landreth, 2002), which is often used to explain the method or effectiveness of play therapy. I use metaphors that my families bring to the therapy room or assist them in discovering a metaphor for themselves. These metaphors become the catalyst for change and self-discovery in so many families, providing an avenue for them to shine and grow in their own unique way.

When children are given the chance to go on a journey of self-discovery within the play therapy room, they are able to discover their own unique voice within that room; a voice that often doesn't include words. They are able to express roles, dynamics, likes and dislikes, and concerns while exploring many ways to learn and express themselves. As a child's language and voice is heard, they begin to embrace their sense of self and competencies. Speaking the language of the child in the family, using their metaphors and their culture to assist in growth is so very powerful.

Clair Mellenthin, MSW, RPT-S

I believe it is of utmost importance to speak the client's language – if we can presume this is the language of play. Play is how children communicate their thoughts, feelings, and emotional experiences. Play crosses the communication gap when there is a language barrier or challenge to the developmental, verbal, or expressed language between adult and child. Play is how children make sense of the world around them, the different relationships in their life, and the challenges they themselves are experiencing or have experienced. Landreth writes,

> Play is a medium of exchange, and restricting children to verbal expression automatically places a barrier to a therapeutic relationship by imposing limitations that in effect say to children, you must come up my level of communication and communicate with words.
>
> (2002, p. 14)

> This is so important to remember, as when it comes to so much of what we experience in life, especially when related to trauma, heartache, grief, and loss, there are no words to adequately verbalize and describe how we feel, what our experiences meant to us, or the impact an event has had in our world. However, when we can play it out and create meaning out of the symbolism and metaphor in front of us, we can find the "words", whether verbal or symbolic, to make sense and develop insight into our experiences.

I think part of "speaking the client's language" comes from allowing the child to direct the process and using the tools and mediums that work best for the client, even if you yourself don't like the toys or game being used. Adults/play therapists can tend to be very restrictive in their therapeutic approach, whether this is a conscious directing by only providing for certain approaches or toys to use or subconscious directing, such as giving the child praise if they "choose" what we like instead of what the child actually desires to do. If we are always directing the play either verbally or through nonverbal methods, the child lacks an opportunity to experience the empowerment and mastery that comes from their own creative process and processing, as they try to please the adult in the room.

When we can join in with the child's play and be attuned to their needs, verbal and/or nonverbal requests, and experiences, we are showing them that they are important and that we *see* them. This is a critical attachment need for every human, and for many children, their play therapy session may be the one place where they can experience feeling accepted for who they are, as they are. Therefore, it is so important to speak *their* language and give them the space and time they need to heal and make sense of their world.

Akiko J. Ohnogi, PsyD

I believe that all mental health professionals, especially play therapists, should prioritize speaking the client's language. Thus, I personally place a lot of importance on it. There is an example that I give play therapy students in explaining the importance of using play when working with children, that seems to help the trainees understand it well. Let's pretend you are fluent in English and speak some French as you grew up in a bilingual environment as a child. As you are the one who needs to understand and be understood, it would be much easier for that to happen if you mainly conversed in English, mixing in French when necessary. How would you feel if your psychotherapist insists on speaking French? How well do you think you would be able to express yourself? Imagine how frustrating it would be trying to convey something in French when you don't have the words or speak it fluently, when it would be so easy to do in your primary language.

For the play therapist to insist on using words to communicate and express a feeling or thought, it is equivalent to your psychotherapist insisting that you speak French when speaking in English would make things much more comfortable, rich, and deeper. Since a play therapist is trained to be able to understand what play behavior is communicating and expressing, it is important that they adapt to using the child's language of play, and not try to make the child speak the adult language of words.

I treat clients from all over the world; thus, our primary spoken language may not necessarily be the same (I am fluent in English and Japanese). With these clients, the use of play becomes especially important. With play, I can discern the child's play theme, as I can see the child's storyline in the play. I would not be able to do this if the child were to use only verbal language. In post-trauma work, it is important to recognize the importance of play as the child's primary source of communication. As trauma temporarily hinders effective use of the "thinking" part of the brain, it is especially important that play be used in the intervention and treatment to directly access the "feeling" part of the brain. For a traumatized brain, their "language" is play, not words (Ohnogi & Drewes, 2016).

Mary Anne Peabody, EdD, RPT-S

I deeply resonate with the work of play therapist Dr. Jodi Mullen (2008) who argues childhood is a culture with distinct status, rules, values, and language. Therefore, if we are to be able to speak our client's language within the clinical context, we must shift our philosophical paradigms and place priority on nonverbal behavior, nonsensical sounds, and the language of play as their preferred mode of expression (Mullen, 2008).

I view play therapists as interpreters of this unique play language. Just as a foreign language interpreter requires specialized knowledge, skills, and competencies, our specialized areas of expertise make us "play language interpreters". Our role becomes one of facilitator, advocate, and educator to ensure the clients preferred language of play is noticed, heard, accepted, and understood. Furthermore, our role extends into interpreting the child's verbal and non-verbal communication for their collateral supports. For parents, this interpreting activity is not simply an exercise in the ability to translate one set of words into another but extends into multifaceted meaning making whereby the play therapist helps parents welcome and understand their child's world and perspective. This awareness can promote opening lines of playful interactions and communication that, in turn, can strengthen the parent-child relationship. Therefore, I place a huge importance on speaking the child's language, and think this is what clearly differentiates play therapists from other therapists.

Dee Ray, PhD, RPT-S

"Toys are children's words, and play is their language" (Landreth, 2012, p. 313). The preceding quote is commonly cited among play therapists as the primary rationale for play therapy. In child-centered play therapy, the relationship is noted as the healing agent for change, not play. Although play has many remarkable positive roles in the lives of children (Schaefer & Drewes, 2014), the child-centered play therapist acknowledges play as the primary language of expression on which to build the therapist-child relationship. Hence, play is the cornerstone of communication in play therapy. Children are in the process of acquiring receptive and spoken language throughout their development; whereas play appears early in childhood as a natural process that is pursued without instruction. Play is the way in which children assimilate and accommodate their worlds (Piaget, 1962).

When adults talk to children, the child is expected to come into the adult's world. But when an adult plays, they move into the child's world. The adult who plays sends the message that the child's world is one of importance and value, and that the child does not have to meet the adult's expectations to be worthy. When I value the child's natural language of play, I send the fundamental message that I do not wish the child were different in some way (Axline, 1947), a powerful, healing message. I often compare speaking the language of play to the speaking of other languages. If I continued to speak Spanish to a client who only speaks Chinese, I would be sending the message that I do not care enough about them to learn their language or communicate with them. It also seems incredibly impractical for me to continue to speak only my language and expect that we are building an effective therapeutic relationship. When adults insist on only talking with children without using the language of play, they send the message that the child is not worthy of the adult's attention to learning their language. Additionally, adults who primarily use words in their language with children are speaking in a language in which a child has limited fluency, an impractical communication practice.

Jessica Stone, PhD, RPT-S

Speaking the client's language is of utmost importance. Entering into their world by *truly* hearing, seeing, and understanding them through their interests and communications (verbal and nonverbal) is a critical cornerstone of any therapeutic process. If we are to understand a person's thought processes, worldview, perceptions, experiences, behaviors, triggers, responses, and more, we must learn their language.

A person's language can be their actual use of verbal and nonverbal communication. Cadence and vernacular are important components of verbal communication. However, a client's interests, what they are attracted to (or not) and why, and what elicits emotional and/or experiential responses are all included in one's language as well. Language in this sense is a mode of communication and expression.

Human beings want to be heard, seen, understood, and valued. If the therapist exhibits an interest in what the client is drawn to, then the message is that the client is important enough to the therapist to remember and invest in the topic. As an example, a young teenaged client once had a slight obsession with a singer, his songs, and all the lyrics. This was not an artist I was familiar with, however, knowing that this person "spoke" to her in ways where she felt included and understood, it was very important that I learn more about this singer. Numerous songs were listened to in the session. Afterward I researched everything I could find about the artist and printed out the lyrics to a number of the teen's favorite songs. The next session was full of in-depth conversations about the findings. This conversation led to revelations about the connections the client had to the expressions. At the conclusion of treatment, the client shared that this was a turning moment in our work together. No one had ever put effort into her interest in this artist, most adults dismissed her in these regards. She said it was then that she knew this time in therapy would be different.

Whatever a client has as an interest, the therapy will benefit from the play therapist investing time and energy into learning more about it. The very act of remembering the interest, learning more, and then working to understand why it is important to the client will be beneficial. Beyond that, some very powerful information and insights will most likely be gleaned from the understandings, and the client will be more willing to allow the therapist further into his/her world.

Daniel Sweeney, PhD, RPT-S

In play therapy, play is considered the child's language and toys are the child's words (Landreth, 2012). Some of my colleagues have argued that play is the only true international language and thus play therapy is inherently cross-cultural. I have done play therapy demonstrations around the world with children who speak other languages, with and without interpreters involved. The nonclinical demonstrations have been successful.

Having said all this, however, it is not my opinion that play therapy can be used with clients who speak a language different from the therapist. Speaking the client's language is crucial. This makes tracking and reflection both possible and effective.

Additionally, since working with parents is so key to the play therapy process, a monolingual English-speaking therapist is at an incredible disadvantage when attempting to work with non–English speaking parents. I have supervised some play therapists who have used the English-speaking children as translators to communicate with their non–English-speaking parent(s). This is fraught with disadvantage, and is potentially damaging to the communication and relationship process. I have had other supervisees who have used interpreters, both in the room or by speaker phone. There are still significant challenges here, the primary one being that the interpreters are trained as interpreters but not as therapists.

Working with interpreters when working with parents can involve multiple challenges. An interpreter can make several mistakes, that would be unknown to the therapist, such as telling a parent not to be upset, "cleaning up" the parent's language (e.g., suppressing curse words), or answering the parent's question without conveying the question to the therapist. Therapists can make mistakes in this process as well, such as failing to even use an interpreter by not recognizing the need, speaking too quickly for the interpreter, or allowing the interpreter to direct a session and not recognizing when a session is going in the wrong direction.

Whereas there is some literature in play therapy about working with multicultural and diverse populations, I am not aware of any literature that discusses the issue of play therapy with non–English-speaking clients. While expressive therapies can be helpful for clients whose primary language is not English, I am personally not in favor of play therapists working with parents unless they are fluent in parent(s)' language.

References

Ashby, J. S., Kottman, T., & DeGraaf, D. (2008). *Active interventions for kids and teens: Adding adventure and fun to counseling.* American Counseling Association.

Axline, V. (1947). *Play therapy.* Ballantine.

Brooks, R. (1981). Creative characters: A technique in child therapy. *Psychotherapy, 18,* 131–139.

Kottman, T., & Ashby, J. S. (2002). Custom designing metaphoric stories for children in play therapy. In. C. E. Schaefer & D. M. Cangelosi (Eds.), *Innovative psychotherapy techniques in child and adolescent therapy* (pp. 133–142). John Wiley & Sons.

Kottman, T., & Meany-Walen, K. (2016). *Partners in play: An Adlerian approach to play therapy* (3rd ed.). American Counseling Association.

Landreth, G. L. (1991). *Play therapy: The art of the relationship*. Accelerated Development Inc. Publishers.

Landreth, G. (2002). *Play therapy: The art of the relationship* (2nd ed.). Routledge.

Landreth, G. (2012). *Play therapy: The art of the relationship* (3rd ed.). Routledge.

McInnes, K. (2019). Being a playful therapist. In P. Ayling, H. Armstrong, & L. G. Clark (Eds.), *Becoming and being a play therapist: Play therapy in practice* (p. 105). Routledge.

Mills, J., & Crowley, R. (2014). *Therapeutic metaphors for children and the child within* (2nd ed.). Routledge.

Mullen, J. A. (2008). Through a cross-cultural lens: How viewing childhood as a distinct culture impacts supervision. In A. A. Drewes & J. A. Mullen (eds.) *Supervision can be playful*. Jason Aronson Publishing.

Ohnogi, A., & Drewes, A. (2016). Play therapy to help school-aged children deal with natural and human-made disasters. In A. Drewes & C. Schaefer (Eds.), *Play therapy in middle childhood* (pp. 33–52). American Psychological Association.

Piaget, J. (1962). *Play, dreams and imitation in childhood*. W.W. Norton & Co.

Schaefer, C., & Drewes, A. (2014). *The therapeutic powers of play: 20 core agents of change* (2nd ed.). Wiley.

8   How Do You Include Parents in the Play Therapy Process?

Jeff Ashby, PhD, RPT-S

Formal parental/caregiver consultation is a regular part of AdPT, and I use it whenever possible (Kottman & Meany-Walen, 2016). One of the basic maxims in AdPT is that if one person in a family has a problem, members of the family all make some contribution to the problem and hence can contribute toward a solution (Kottman, personal communication, November 25, 2019). As a result, I try to engage parents in all four phases of AdPT. In the first phase, developing an egalitarian relationship, I ask parents to openly share about what is going on in their family and their perspective about the presenting problem, the family dynamics, and any past intervention strategies that have been tried. In the second phase, exploring the client's lifestyle, I meet with parents to solicit their perceptions of the client's lifestyle, the parents' own lifestyles, and the interaction between their lifestyles and the child's lifestyle.

In the first two phases of therapy, I formulate hypotheses about the client's lifestyle and about the parenting interactions that might contribute to the client's distress and those that might help facilitate positive change. In the third and fourth phases of play therapy, helping clients gain insight into their lifestyle and reorientation/reeducation, I try to facilitate parents' consideration of new ways of thinking about their child and new strategies for interacting with their child. In the consultation process, I also consider the parents' lifestyles in the design of the consultation (Kottman & Ashby, 1999). As parents gain some insight into their child's lifestyles, they can also see how the interaction with their own lifestyles might be setting a context for the presenting problem.

Throughout parental consultation, I try to listen reflectively. As I am able to build a relationship with parents/caregivers, I may engage in didactic teaching to help parents/caregivers gain insight into their child (e.g., goals of misbehavior). I may also help parent/caregivers build parenting skills such as structuring, setting logical consequences, setting up routines, and offering positive and constructive feedback to their child.

While not the focus of this question, I also highly value teacher consultation. Just as parents have a significant impact on children, so too do teachers.

If I can enlist teachers, through effective consultation, the child and classroom benefit. I conceptualize my role, as Kottman (2011) identified it, as "partner, encourager, and teacher with parents, teachers and siblings". (p. 97).

Robert Jason Grant, EdD, RPT-S

I often include parents in my play therapy work. Many of my clients are children and adolescents with development disorders. Because of this, I implement AutPlay therapy (Grant, 2017) which is an integrative family play therapy approach. In this approach, parents are considered cochange agents in the therapy process. Parents are in the play sessions with the child – learning, playing, and experiencing together. Formally, parents are taught how to implement special play times and play therapy interventions at home with their child. These interventions are typically focused on skill developments that have been identified and established as treatment goals. Parents continue to be involved until treatment goals have been met and therapy is terminated.

I also use filial therapy (VanFleet, 2014). Some parents and children enter therapy with a very strained relationship. Parents may be dealing with high levels of stress and frustration with their child or their child's condition and subsequent behaviors. In these cases, I would begin therapy with filial therapy, and once that has been completed, I would move into AutPlay therapy. I have found filial therapy to be very effective for improving the parent/child relationship and preparing parents to move into a more parent-implemented therapy such as AutPlay therapy. The National Autism Center's National Standards Project (2015) identified 27 evidence-based practices for working with children with autism. One of the evidenced-based practices is parent training and parent-implemented intervention. There are multiple play therapy approaches that actively include parents or family members. Besides AutPlay and filial therapy, child-parent relationship therapy (2019), Theraplay (2010), and general family play therapy interventions exist. Any of these approaches would meet the requirements of the evidence-based parent-implemented intervention practice for working with children with autism.

Occasionally, I might forgo a more formal family play therapy approach. In these situations, I would still have some type of check-in process established with parents. This might be checking in at the beginning of each session to get updates or information they may want to tell me, or I might have a parent check-in session established every fourth or fifth session. In some cases, I provide a feedback form that parents can complete and e-mail back to me before the child's session. How I involve a parent varies depending on the parent and what seems to work best for them. Some cautions when working with parents include avoiding parents "taking over" the child's session (using the child's time to talk about their own issues) and trying to talk with me after the child's session is over (updates should happen at the beginning of the session). I have found that both situations can be very negative to the therapy process, especially for the child.

Heidi Gerard Kaduson, PhD, RPT-S

I attempt to involve parents in the process of play therapy but generally not in the playroom with the child. This certainly depends on the specific issues of the child, parents, family, and so on. I do two intakes on different days. One intake is for caregivers only, where they respond to many questions I would have regarding the history and current situation of the child. On another day, I meet with the child only in the playroom, and based on the information I received from parents, I provide the type of environment the child needs (no drawing is required if there are fine motor difficulties, no loud music if the child has sensory integration problems, etc.). After the play intake with the child, I send detailed notes to the caregivers, describing exactly what was done and how their child responded. That is the only time I send an e-mail describing the playtime, since I meet with parents regularly before sessions with the child.

There are many valid reasons to use filial therapy (Guerney, 2003), Theraplay (Jernberg & Booth, 2001) or other structured parent involvement for play therapy, but it must be matched to the family dynamics, the child's disorder, and the limitations of the situation the family is in. For children on the autistic spectrum, many can benefit from these parent-child interaction models of play therapy. For separation anxiety I would have parents bring the child into the playroom, sit on a child-height chair near the door and say nothing and provide no engagement with their child. If I am able to engage the child, I would have the parents ask where the restroom is and try to naturally leave the room. In most other cases, I would spend 10 minutes alone with the parent in my office (after child is comfortable by himself in playroom) and give a parent training intervention to help assist them in parenting their specific child. I recommend if there are negative events that happen at home, they can leave that information on my confidential voice mail or e-mail with HIPPA restrictions in place. Typically, after the first meeting, I would have parents record the child's positive behavior in a "Good Behavior Book" (Kaduson, 2020, 2000). This helps to include the positive behaviors of the child rather than trying to work only with the negative in mind.

Jennifer Lefebre, PsyD, RPT-S

I involve parents in the play therapy process in many different ways. With some families, the primary focus is family play therapy, as the "client" is truly the family system. In these cases, family play therapy is focused on attachment, regulation, connection, and competency. I use variations of Theraplay® integrated with strategies from EMDR when working in these systems. For other children, family sessions are integrated on a monthly basis in addition to individual therapy. In these cases, there are often individual needs of the child and a smaller family component, and family sessions are more prescriptive or strategic in nature. With some children (typically not younger than 12), parents are included via consult sessions and less frequent family therapy. I don't have a one size fits all approach, but I believe parents are vital to the therapy process and I integrate them in as many different ways as I can.

One thing I do with all families I work with, regardless of age, diagnostics, or presenting problems, is find ways they can play well together. Traditions, cooking meals, games, routines and chores, outdoor activities, music, and sports – these are ways that families can learn about the therapeutic powers of play in terms of how play is already positively affecting their lives. This manner of psychoeducation nicely leads to the creation of new adventures for the family, as a means to increase attachment and competencies. When I explain the importance of these activities as an avenue for change and growth for the family as a whole, most members seem to engage and are excited to tell me their adventure of the week, even if it was a treasure hunt for a can of peas in the grocery store.

Clair Mellenthin, MSW, RPT-S

I try to involve parents early on in the play therapy process, as I believe wholeheartedly that lasting change can only happen if we help parents to change and allow for healing to happen. We can't expect the least powerful, most vulnerable person in the family system to be the one to make a lasting change happen. We need to involve the person/people who do have the power to make changes and to help the system activate healing. Depending on the attachment needs of the child and family system as a whole, the involvement of parents in the therapeutic process varies. With every client, I meet with parents (without the child) during the first session in order to candidly discuss the parents' concerns and the developmental history of their child, and to assess the parent's attachment history and parenting strategies they employ at home. When working with a family whose parents have divorced and they are unable to meet together, I will schedule a separate appointment for each parent. This must be completed before I will work with the child. In cases of divorce, each parent must also sign a nonlitigation and custody dispute contract that states they will not involve the therapist in custody disputes or court hearings, use their child's play therapy sessions in court, or request the clinical notes of the therapy sessions. I schedule parent consultations every 4–6 weeks, where parents and I will meet without the child present to discuss ongoing concerns, treatment goals, and teach attachment-centered parenting techniques.

My goal with every child client is to help their parent(s) or caregiver to become a resource to the child, by strengthening and repairing the attachment between them. Therefore, their involvement in some capacity is critical. For some families, parents are ready and able to attend parent-child play therapy sessions from the beginning of treatment. These families tend to be mostly securely attached and have a strong relationship in place. Other parents may need to do their own therapeutic work or attend a parenting program before they are in a place emotionally to be able to join in their child's therapy process.

My expectations of parents include the following: if they are in the play-room, they are active participants in their child's play therapy sessions. I don't allow parents to come into the session to passively observe or record their child's play therapy session (yes, this has been attempted in the past!). I have found that the majority of parents are grateful for this opportunity, even if it initially brings up feelings of fear and vulnerability. As we create healing in the attachment relationship between the parent and child, we can help to build a secure foundation for the family to stand on.

Akiko J. Ohnogi, PsyD

I include caregivers in a child and/or adolescent play therapy treatment with-out exception. I do this by scheduling parent consultations, and parents are asked to participate in parent-child play therapy sessions. Parent involvement is especially important for young children when addressing attachment issues, and if parents and child have both experienced a traumatic event. Parents and the child are present in sessions during most of the treatment process.

I begin treatment with a parent-only consultation session before meeting with the child and schedule subsequent parent consultation sessions every 4–6 weeks. I will meet more often if necessary or if requested by the parent. I also check in with parents, with the child present, at the beginning of ev-ery session. I ask that both parents come to the initial parent consultation session (when both parents are involved in the child's life together) and if only one parent is available, I will meet with the other parent at a different consultation session.

At least one parent must always accompany the child to every session and stay for the duration of the scheduled session, even if it is simply waiting in the waiting room. If the parent wishes to discuss something, I will schedule a sep-arate consultation session, and do not take away time from the child's session.

I only accept clients whose parents are willing to participate in treatment. I do not see clients if the nanny brings the child, a parent drops off the child and runs an errand, and so on. For children who are living in an orphanage, I ask that their main caregiver at the orphanage participate in the sessions as would a parent. For children who are in the care of other adults (grandparents, aunts and uncles, etc.), I ask that these caregivers participate in the sessions as would a parent. For children whose parents are divorced but are able to do things with the child's best interest in mind (even if the parents' relationship with each other is acrimonious), I will see the child with each parent in attendance separately. The schedule of which parent participates at what time will depend on their schedules and motivation, and the effect on treatment progress. The type, frequency, and duration of parent-child play sessions are dependent on the necessity and/or usefulness of including playing together in the treatment, for both the parent and child/adolescent.

Mary Anne Peabody, EdD, RPT-S

Including parents in the play therapy process is one of the distinctive elements of my practice. I believe parental participation engagement is often pivotal as to whether therapy is or is not successful (Peabody, 2020). I agree with the words of Clair Mellenthin (2019) when she states, "excluding parents in the child's therapeutic journey is like trying to solve a jigsaw puzzle with only half of the pieces" (p. 1). In the cases where parent involvement is not possible or contraindicated, I will see the child with minimal or no parental involvement, but this is extremely rare for me. I also believe if we give our skills away to parents, not only does the identified child client benefit, but our therapeutic reach grows exponentially.

Borrowing from Adlerian play therapy, I use play-based approaches in my parent consultation meetings (Kottman & Meany-Walen, 2018). I believe parents need to both understand and experience the therapeutic powers of play themselves (Peabody, in press). As a prescriptive play therapist, if the best treatment available for a specific client's issues involves one of the parent-child play therapy approaches I have been trained in, I may utilize child-parent relationship therapy (Bratton et al., 2006); filial play therapy (Vanfleet, 2005) or family play therapy (Gil, 2015).

Finally, I often refer parents to Pam Leo's book *Connecting through Parenting* (2011) that is built on the premise of connecting before correcting. She challenges adults to think about interactions with children and to contemplate if our words or actions will strengthen or weaken the connection. Another book I frequently give to parents is *Playful Parenting* by Lawrence Cohen (2001). Cohen situates play in parenting practices to help build connections and teaches parents strategies to enter the emotional world of their world. By teaching parents about the role of positive emotions when they engage in playful interactions with their children, I feel I make a significant contribution.

Dee Ray, PhD, RPT-S

Children come with parents. Children exist because a person became a parent. Hence, working with parents is a key process of play therapy. I include parents in the process in several different ways. Prior to beginning the play therapy relationship with the child, I meet with the parent to conduct a thorough interview regarding the child's background, developmental history, and presenting concerns. In this interview, I seek to build a relationship with the parent in which they feel understood, accepted, and cared for. I believe that the essential relational conditions required for my relationship with the child are also required for my relationship with the parent. As we embark on the play therapy process, I typically facilitate a family play session within the initial phase of the play therapy relationship in order to assess family dynamics and relationships. In this session, I will often conduct a family art assessment (Landgarten, 1987) or family puppet interview (Irwin & Malloy, 1994).

The purpose of the initial family play session is to increase my empathic understanding of the child's world, engage parents in the play therapy process, and develop a systemic treatment plan. Based on the child's process in play therapy sessions, the initial parent interview, and the initial family play session, I will determine how the parent should be involved for optimal progress. Some parents need education and skills while other parents may just need emotional support for their parenting. Some parents need frequent parent consultations while other parents only need to meet once a month. Some parent-child dyads are better served by family play sessions, while some children are in need of their own individual therapy. Some parents need to be in their own therapy in addition to or instead of their child. I attempt to map out systemic plans based on the unique nature of each family.

Typically, I work with parents in a consultation role. From a child-centered play therapy approach, I consider the child to be my client and the parent a systemic partner. Under normal circumstances, I meet with parents every 3–5 play therapy sessions in order to check in with them about events at home, discuss progress in play therapy, teach parenting skills, and practice skills (Ray, 2011). Research has shown play therapy to show greater positive effects when parents are involved in therapy (Bratton et al., 2005; Lin & Bratton, 2015). My experience is that parent investment in play therapy directly influences the progress of play therapy. However, it should be noted that child-centered play therapy has been shown to be effective when parents are not part of the process (e.g., Cheng & Ray, 2016; Ray et al., 2013; Wilson & Ray, 2018). I believe the finding that children demonstrate progress in play therapy without parent involvement is notable because we, as play therapists, often do not have access to or willingness from parents to be a part of the process. Yet we can be confident that although therapy may be limited from reaching full potential without parent involvement, children are able to meaningfully address their struggles when provided a therapeutic environment only for them.

Jessica Stone, PhD, RPT-S

Parents and caregivers can be very important components of the play therapy process. Their involvement may be necessary to meet the treatment goals. Typically, my focus is the sacred protection of the child's session time, and the inclusion of others would be for very specific therapeutic purposes.

The initial consult does not include the child under the age of 12, and any special circumstance of initial inclusion would be determined on a case-by-case basis. The consult for the child under the age of 12 does not include the child initially for several reasons. There might be topics the parent would not want to discuss in front of the child or, in some cases, there are parents who would discuss things I would not want discussed in front of a young child. Caregiver boundaries can be difficult/impossible to predict prior to the intake. I also do not want the child exposed to a number of clinicians if the parents are evaluating the best fit for their family. Until it is known that I will be the clinician, there is no reason for the child to meet/be exposed to numerous people and offices. The intake process continues when the child comes in to determine the next level of "good fit".

People who are over the age of 12 are asked to attend the intake. Most people do not want to think of others sitting around talking about them when they are not present. In people over the age of 12, the result of an intake without them could hinder the rapport building process. In these consults, the caregivers are included for the first half of the intake and then they are asked to wait in the waiting room while the client and I talk for a bit about their desires and goals for coming in.

After the initial consult appointment(s), parental involvement is either on an as-needed basis or in regular increments, depending on the treatment goals. At times, a parent will be invited into session with the client's assent. This is predominately done when there is a rupture in the relationship and either I need to assess this rupture to determine the next phases of the treatment plan, or connections need to be made within session to further the existing therapeutic goals. At times, families are referred out for family therapy if more than one or two family meetings are needed. I typically do not assume the role of the family therapist in addition to the individual therapist as I feel it has a high potential to negatively impact the individual dynamic. Periodic caregiver meetings or family sessions can be invaluable for further information gathering, assessments, role modeling, parental consultation, clarifying treatment goals, and setting or altering the treatment plan.

Daniel Sweeney, PhD, RPT-S

I have supervised play therapists who find working with parents to be a bewildering part of the play therapy process. Parents must, however, be a part of the play therapy process in order for that process to be successful. I agree with Ray (2011), who maintains,

> Play therapists often cite working with parents or guardians as the most challenging aspect of counseling with children. To have access to working with children, play therapists must forge a positive and collaborative relationship with their parents. When parents feel alienated, blamed, or ignored in the therapy process, they will typically terminate services.
>
> (p. 141)

Ray (2011) goes on to make several points regarding play therapists' attitudes that can provide a basis for a collaborative relationship with parents:

- *Respect for the parent's role.* Play therapists will be much more effective if they recognize the role of the parent as the most important relationship in the child's life.

- *Respect for the parent's knowledge of the child.* Even the most neglectful of parents often possess intimate knowledge of the child and the child's development needed by the play therapist to enhance the effectiveness of the therapist.
- *Affection for the parent as a person.* In working with children who have experienced traumatic parenting or a lack of parenting, play therapists may often become less likely to present as caring and nurturing to parents – play therapists will be more effective if they can overcome such feelings and work toward a true care for the parent.
- *Patience.* The relationship between parent and play therapist is enhanced when the play therapist maintains an attitude of patience.
- *Clear focus on child as the client.* In the model presented in this book, the child is the client and parents are seen as systemic partners in therapy. (pp. 142–143)

I begin the process of play therapy by meeting with the parent(s) without the child present. I want parents to meet me, receive some information about the play therapy process, and have the parents explain the presenting issue. This explanation is often a rather intense and pejorative description of the child – which is quite understandable, considering the stress that the parent(s) are experiencing. However, I do not want this negative "download" to occur in the presence of the child. This could be damaging in and of itself, and I do not want the child to see me aligned as just one more adult with a negative perspective on the child. I briefly consult with the parents every session (outside of the hearing of the child), and set up half- or full-session consults as needed.

My primary choice in working with parents is through parent training – using my preference of filial therapy (Guerney, 1964; Landreth & Bratton, 2020). Since my experience has been that a large percentage of child referrals are for issues related to noncompliance, I consider the presenting issue to be a parent-child problem as opposed to a child problem. Thus, parent training is frequently my preference. This is obviously dependent on the willingness and availability of the parent(s). Even in cases of a trauma presentation, I prefer to transition to filial therapy training at an appropriate time.

References

Bratton, S. C., Landreth, G. L., Kellam, T., & Blackard, S. R. (2006). *Child parent relationship therapy (CPRT) treatment manual: A 10-session filial therapy model for training parents.* Routledge/Taylor & Francis Group.

Bratton, S., Ray, D., Rhine, T., & Jones, L. (2005). The efficacy of play therapy with children: A meta-analytic review of treatment outcomes. *Professional Psychology: Research and Practice, 36,* 376–390. doi:10.1037/0735-7028.36.4.376.

Cheng, Y., & Ray, D. (2016). Child centered group play therapy: Impact on social emotional assets of Kindergarten children. *Journal for Specialists in Group Work, 41*, 209–237. doi:10.1080/01933922.2016.1197350.

Cohen, L. (2001). *Playful parenting: An exciting new approach to raising children that will help you nurture close connections, behavior problems, and encourage confidence.* Random House.

Gill, E. (2015). *Play in family therapy.* Guilford Press.

Grant, R. J. (2017). *AutPlay therapy for children and adolescents on the autism spectrum: A behavioral play-based approach.* Routledge.

Guerney, B. G. (1964). Filial therapy: Description and rationale. *Journal of Consulting Psychology, 28*(4), 303–310.

Guerney, L. (2003). Filial play therapy. In C. E. Schaefer (Ed.), *Foundations of play therapy* (pp. 99–142). Wiley.

Irwin, E., & Malloy, E. (1994). Family puppet interview. In C. Schaefer & L. Carey (Eds.), *Family play therapy* (pp. 21–33). Rowman & Littlefield.

Landgarten, H. (1987). *Family art psychotherapy: A clinical guide and casebook.* Brunner/Mazel.

Landreth, G. L., & Bratton, S. (2020). *Child-parent relationship therapy (CPRT): An evidence-based 10-session filial therapy model* (2nd ed.). Routledge.

Leo, P. (2011). *Connection parenting.* Wyatt-MacKenzie Publishing, Inc.

Lin, Y., & Bratton, S. (2015). A meta-analytic review of child-centered play therapy approaches. *Journal of Counseling and Development, 93*, 45–58. doi:10.1002/j.1556-6676.2015.00180.x.

Jernberg. A. & Booth, P. B. (2001). *Theraplay: Helping parents and children build better relationships through attachment-based play* (2nd ed.). Jossey-Bass.

Kaduson, H. G. (2000). Structured short-term play therapy or children with attention-deficit hyperactivity disorder. In H. G. Kaduson & C. E. Schaefer (Eds.), *Short-term play therapy for children* (pp. 105–143). Guilford Press.

Kaduson, H. G. (2020). Play therapy for children with attention-deficit hyperactivity disorder. In H. G. Kaduson, D. Cangelosi, & C. E. Schaefer (Eds.), *Prescriptive play therapy: Tailoring interventions for specific childhood problems* (pp. 161–177). Guilford Press.

Kottman, T. (2011). Adlerian play therapy. In C. Schaefer (Ed.), *Foundations of play therapy* (2nd ed., pp. 87–104). Wiley.

Kottman, T., & Ashby, J. S. (1999). Using Adlerian personality priorities to custom design parental consultation. *International Journal of Play Therapy, 8*, 77–92.

Kottman, T., & Meany-Walen, K. (2016). *Partners in play: An Adlerian approach to play therapy* (3rd ed.). American Counseling Association.

Kottman, T. & Meany-Walen, K. (2018). *Doing play therapy.* Guilford Press.

Mellenthin, C. (2019). *Attachment centered play therapy.* Routledge.

National Standards Project (2015). National Autism Center at May Institute. https://www.nationalautismcenter.org/national-standards-project/.

Peabody, M. A. (2020). Parent involvement in children's game play: Accelerating the therapeutic impact. In J. Stone & C. E. Schaefer (Eds.), *Game play: The use of games with children and adolescents* (3rd ed., pp. 9–25). Wiley.

Peabody, M. A. (in press). Building understanding in parent consultation brick by brick. *Play Therapy.*

Ray, D. (2011). *Advanced play therapy: Essential conditions, knowledge, and skills for child practice.* Routledge.

Ray, D., Stulmaker, H., Lee, K., & Silverman, W. (2013). Child centered play therapy and impairment: Exploring relationships and constructs. *International Journal of Play Therapy, 22*, 13–27.

VanFleet, R. (2005). *Filial therapy: Strengthening parent-child relationships through play* (2nd ed.). Professional Resource Press.

VanFleet, R. (2014). *Filial Therapy: strengthening parent-child relationships through play* (3rd ed.). Professional Resource Press.

Wilson, B., & Ray, D. (2018). Child centered play therapy: Aggression, empathy, and self-regulation. *Journal of Counseling & Development, 96*, 399–409.

9 What Is the Importance of Regulation in Your Play Therapy Work; How Is It Best Achieved?

Jeff Ashby, PhD, RPT-S

Emotional regulation is an important part of my play therapy work. While there is some disagreement about the exact definition of regulation, there is consensus that self-regulation includes skills that develop from early childhood, are related to a variety of aspects of social competence and maladjustment, and can be adversely affected by traumatic stress (e.g., Eisenberg & Sulik, 2012; Hebert et al., 2018). Early within my play therapy work with clients, I assess the child's capacity to emotionally self-regulate. Specifically, I am assessing what Eisenberg, Hofer, and Vaughan (2007) define as "the processes used to manage and change if, when, and how (e.g., how intensely) one experiences emotions and emotion-related motivational and physiological states, as well as how emotions are expressed behaviorally" (p. 288).

In the first two phases of my work with children (building an egalitarian relationship and assessing the child's lifestyle), and through initial parent and teacher consultation, I work to understand the client's strengths and assets and areas where skills, like emotional regulation, might be helpful. In stages three and four (helping the child gain insight into lifestyle and reorientation/reeducation), I may design interventions to help build emotional regulation skills. In designing these interventions, I try to stay mindful of the importance of scaffolding the skills and behaviors I am trying to build (Vygotsky, 1978). A number of studies (e.g., Eisenberg et al., 2010) have suggested that self-regulation skills can be strengthened and taught with practice opportunities across contexts and support. Through creative interventions, I can vary the context for developing and practicing these skills.

Coregulation of the client is another important aspect of my work in play therapy. As Sbarra and Hazan (2008) note, healthy people may often rely on others to coregulate their level of arousal and children who have not experienced this coregulation from parents or other caregivers are less likely to develop the ability to self-regulate. In my play therapy work with clients, I attempt to coregulate the client by being consistently warm and responsive in my interactions and model expression of thoughts and feelings. Coregulation of the client is particularly important in the context of parent and teacher consultation. As I am able to help parents and teachers build the skills to coregulate the client (often after helping them build self-regulation skills), the client is offered additional contexts to practice self-regulation and limit the behaviors and interactions that are hindering their success (e.g., tantrums, aggression, acting out).

Robert Jason Grant, EdD, RPT-S

Much of my work focuses on regulation. The concepts of addressing dysregulation, learning self-regulation, and improving emotional regulation ability are typical treatment goals. The populations I work with (developmental disorders) are prone to dysregulation struggles. Many children with autism and related conditions struggle with staying regulated and being able to self-regulate. Children with developmental disorders can become dysregulated quickly and easily and for a variety of reasons which include an inability to understand and modulate emotions, sensory processing struggles, lack of social skills, and inability to adjust to changes and unexpected happenings. Additionally, these children do not understand what is happening within their system and lack knowledge on how to regulate. Much of the dysregulation leads to unwanted behavior that can create further problems for the child.

I often establish a regulation program that can be implemented at home and ideally at school. This program consists of several play interventions that help the child regulate their system. Typically, the child participates in these regulation interventions for approximately 20 minutes a day or every other day. The interventions are chosen based on what the child enjoys playing and what seems to help his or her system to regulate. Many of the regulation play interventions focus on relaxation, sensory input, and movement. This program has been helpful in decreasing dysregulation and thus behavior issues and helping children learn to self-regulate. It is important to note that the play therapist should try to discover what is creating the dysregulation struggles for the child. Is it a sensory processing issue, an inability to recognize and manage emotions, a social skill deficit, high anxiety levels, a combination of factors, and so on? Discovering what is creating the dysregulation will guide what play therapy interventions to use to help the child regulate.

Heidi Gerard Kaduson, Ph.D., RPT-S

If this is about self-regulation, then it depends on the child. Limits are necessary; there is no therapy without limits, but I believe in training a child to have more regulation through play and not just limit setting. I have worked with children with Attention-deficit Hyperactivity Disorder for my entire career. It became clear to me early on that just going through the motions of teaching self-control or self-regulation didn't work well with this population. As I engaged the children more in play, through cognitive-behavioral play therapy (Knell, 1993) and release play therapy (Kaduson, 2015), it became clear that when children feel what self-regulation is like – and they know it in their bodies – they are able to have more self-regulation when we praise and encourage the same.

For ADHD children to gain self-control, they must first feel it to know what it is like. Just talking about what self-control is doesn't always translate into behavior change for children. Therefore, several games can be used for this purpose such as *Rebound* (Mattel), a game that uses ball-bearing pieces to slide on the board, hit two rubber bands and then land in the target zone. Most children with ADHD start this game by flinging the piece very hard, which gets them no points, and the piece can sometimes leave the board altogether. The therapist tells children to practice. This practicing time allows for the assessment of the child's ability to show self-restraint. When the therapist sees that restraint – however small it is – she praises the child by saying, "Now that was self-control". It may take more than five trials before the self-control is seen, but ADHD children are very competitive, so as long as they feel they are getting better at the game, they stick with it. Strategic board games are also used for the child to exhibit self-regulation by taking turns, waiting, and so on, and the therapist praises and encourages more of it. Children feel better when they are self-regulated and, certainly they receive less criticism if they are able to generalize skill gains to home and school settings.

Jennifer Lefebre, PsyD, RPT-S

Regulation is the foundation for most of my work, both clinical and in trainings. I utilize components of SMART: sensory motor arousal regulation treatment (Warner, Cook, Westcott & Koomar, 2011) and attachment, regulation, and competency (ARC) framework (Blaustein & Kinniburgh, 2010) to begin to coregulate and establish some moderate self-regulation. SMART blends connection with others and movement in order to regulate arousal states by utilizing sensory equipment (i.e., weighted blankets, balance beams, fitness balls, large cushions, swings) with shared embodied play to support children's natural ways of regulating their bodies and their emotions, thus facilitating attachment-building and allowing for embodied processing of their traumatic experiences. ARC provides a theoretical framework for working with youth and families who have experienced significant trauma. ARC strengthens attachments by focusing on supporting the caregiving system and creating trauma-informed responses and assists children in self-regulating by increasing skills and awareness in all aspects of their internal experience. ARC also increases empowerment and choice-making skills, as well as an understanding of self and competencies.

A child's dysregulation is noticeable if they are over- or underresponsive to sensory input in ANY of the sensory systems (Ogden & Minton, 2000). While some children may have a high threshold for comfortably managing and responding adaptively to various degrees of arousal, others may present with a limited and constricted capacity to tolerate them. When a child is overresponsive or hypersensitive (i.e., hyperresponsive), they become hypervigilant about the slightest sensations or interoceptive cues (i.e., hunger, thirst, bathroom needs, temperature), leading to sensory overload, anxiety, or pain. A child who is underresponsive or hyposensitive (i.e., hyporesponsive) may not realize they are hungry or thirsty until they are completely starving or dehydrated, or they may have frequent accidents because they do not recognize the need to use the restroom, often needing a large amount of input in order to recognize the type of sensory information their brain is receiving. Embodied play therapy engages the sensory motor systems (e.g., vestibular, proprioceptive, tactile) to facilitate emotional, psychological, and relational regulation and repair.

So, why is the ability to regulate important in play therapy work? When our regulatory and sensory systems are working together, we have the *window of tolerance*, a concept that was brought up by Dan Siegel (1999), which highlights the capacity to tolerate various intensities of arousal, meaning you are able to perceive, process, and react to sensory stimuli and information in a timely manner (Ogden & Minton, 2000; van der Kolk, 2014). A child's window of tolerance needs to be widened for all emotional states (both positive and negative) in order for healing to occur. Children – all people – need to be available for positive relational connection, as well as to be able to handle difficult emotions, so that healthy development can proceed.

The somatosensory experiences in many play activities have been viewed as the neurological foundations for creativity, abstract thought, prosocial behavior, and expressive language (Perry, 2006), as these experiences engage the subcortical, cortical, and attachment neural pathways to integrate psychological, emotional, and behavioral regulation. Play therapy does not rely on language or cognitive awareness as an entry point. When we follow the child's lead (while cultivating safety) and engage in fully embodied participatory play with the child, we restore the capacity for growth and healing. Through the power of play, children will feel safer and become more regulated due to the patterned, repetitive, and rhythmic input that is available during child-directed free play and somatosensory play.

Clair Mellenthin, MSW, RPT-S

A child who isn't regulated is unable to fully engage in a therapeutic process. A child who presents as dysregulated may be experiencing a host of treatment issues such as trauma, anxiety, autism, sensory processing disorder, and ADHD, to name a few. It is important to use "bottom up" approaches when trying to alleviate dysregulation, as this is a neurobiological process occurring. An easy way to remember this is to think of the hand model of the brain that Daniel Siegel popularized. We first need to calm the brain stem (body movement), moving to the primal brain (limbic system), and lastly address the prefrontal cortex (thinking, planning, semantics). I find that for most children, if I remain in a calm state, exhibiting deep, slow breathing, this can help to contain the internal chaos as they begin mirroring this themselves. For other children, we may need to do more guided regulation work, utilizing big, deep breaths or turning off the lights (my playroom has a wall of windows facing outdoors, allowing for daylight to filter in so that the child and therapist are not in complete darkness), laying on the floor on big comfortable pillows, and looking out at the mountains outside. As the child's body is able to calm down, their breathing becomes deep and slow. This is a visible external shift that takes place when regulation occurs. It is only then that it would be appropriate to begin talking through or about their thoughts, feelings, or behaviors.

At times, I will employ and teach an EMDR process called Butterfly Hugs. This is a regulation strategy that a child, caregiver, and therapist can utilize when needed. The child crosses their arms across their chest and hooks their two thumbs together, creating a butterfly. The hands are placed just below the collarbone, with the fingers resting either on the shoulders or upper arms, wherever it feels most comfortable. The child can then slowly begin tapping their arms, left to right and breathing deeply and slowly. Some individuals also prefer to rock back and forth gently while they are tapping. When there is a healthy relationship between the parent and child, this can be a very nurturing way to facilitate coregulation as they either sit side by side and employ this simultaneously or the parent can sit behind the child and gently hug them while slowly tapping the child's arms back and forth.

Akiko J. Ohnogi, PsyD

I feel that the regulation of everyone involved in play therapy is very important, whether it be the child, parents, and/or the play therapist. If someone in the session is dysregulated, it makes it extremely difficult to be able to conduct successful play therapy treatment. In terms of treatment and regulation of the child client, I assess the lowest impacted brain level at the beginning of the session, and if necessary, I start with interventions to regulate their brain before conducting any other type of intervention. I also assess the parents and myself throughout the session, adjusting interventions and interactions as necessary so that everyone's regulation is maintained and any dysregulation is effectively addressed.

As I work a lot with natural disaster trauma patients, I need to incorporate several interventions targeted toward regulating the brainstem, especially in the beginning of treatment to regulate their traumatized brains. In order for treatment of the child/adolescent to go well, I also need to do this with their parents if they have also been traumatized in the same disaster (not to treat the parents but to regulate them so that they can be supportive of their child's treatment).

The following are two examples of activities I have found especially helpful in teaching regulation strategies to children and parents:

- *Happy Breath* – An imagery-based deep breathing technique where the child breathes deeply in through the nose and out through the mouth. When breathing in, the child imagines feelings of happiness, excitement, and calmness coursing through their body. When breathing out, the child imagines feelings of sad, mad, and scared going out of various parts of the body.

- *Stick and String* – (also known as "Cooked and Uncooked Spaghetti"). The child tenses up his or her muscles and imagines their body to be hard and immobile like a stick. The child relaxes his or her muscles and should be flexible and floppy like a string.
- *Carpet Hug* – Invite the children to lie down on a carpet, touching the carpet with their whole body. Count to see how long the children can be still without speaking. Count out loud. Stop at 100 or when the children have calmed their breathing and activity level.

Mary Anne Peabody, EdD, RPT-S

Regulation starts with me. My own regulation requires me to be consciously aware of my breathing, heartrate, and the realization of the range of feelings bubbling within me. Having a sense of self includes a strong awareness of the many changes that take place within my neurophysiological system and how I manage the intensity of whatever is happening within me. This self-awareness and ability to manage is what I strive for not only in my play therapy work but actually in all other aspects of my professional and personal being.

Specific to children, I believe one of the greatest contributions to the play therapy field during my lifetime is the neurobiological and interpersonal perspectives that weave together our understanding of attachment, trauma, and the ability to regulate (Badenoch, 2008; Perry & Szalavitz, 2006; Siegal, 2012; van der Kolk, 2014). I believe for children, coregulation with significant adults comes before self-regulation. If a child has not had consistent and regular models of how to handle big emotions, and/or has experienced trauma, or is born with or acquired physiological changes that makes regulation difficult, coregulation preceding self-regulation is going to be consistently needed.

I am a fan of Paris Goodyear-Brown's prop-based playful relaxation exercises that I often use to structure the beginning and ending of sessions (Goodyear-Brown, 2010). These may include materials housed permanently in the playroom such as a sand tray, or specific items that I use only during the structuring activity such as (balancing peacock feathers, guided imagery scripts, or yoga position cards). I believe as a therapist, I have a responsibility to directly teach, model, and facilitate skills that help with regulation including limit setting, emotionally responsive interactions and language, and feeling recognition. Therefore, I use a multiplicity of play-based stress inoculation strategies with the child and the parent in the play therapy sessions and often recommend parents continue the strategies at home between our sessions.

Finally, as both a seasoned play therapist and a mature adult, I recognize my humanness and imperfections. It is a humbling realization that there are times when my ability to regulate my own emotions is challenging. I believe these moments are important lessons, if I can remain open to learning. I often reflect on, when I struggle, the state of the parents of our clients and the clients themselves. Many are feeling exhausted or discouraged by the time they find us and as they attempt to learn new skills. We need to stay compassionate with others and with ourselves.

Dee Ray, PhD, RPT-S

Emotional and physical regulation is the goal for the child but also for the therapist. We often only think of regulation in terms of the child and what the play therapist needs to do to help regulate the child. However, I find that the therapist's level of self-regulation has the most influence over the child's ability to regulate in play therapy. As a play therapist, I need to operate from a high level of self-awareness about how my current state-of-being is affecting my emotional and physical regulation. I tend to identify as a person who is prone to anxiety. If I am dealing with a considerable amount of stress, either personally or professionally, I notice that my body is tense, my jaw is tight, my heartbeat is faster, and I am overly alert. In this state, I am likely to enter a play session dysregulated from the beginning which will affect the child and my relationship with the child. Hence, I need to engage in regular self-awareness and respond with self-care to ensure that I am regulated in my general day-to-day state.

At other times, I may be in a general state of regulation, but I may possibly be affected by some children in play sessions in which they are overly aggressive, rejecting, chaotic, or exhibit other behaviors that are challenging. If I become dysregulated in response to a child's dysregulation, I am likely to respond in a way that intensifies the child's inability to regulate self. At these times, I have a few techniques that I use. I will notice that my heartbeat is beating faster or I am breathing unevenly and allow this observation to come into my awareness. I will take a brief second or two to be mindful before I make any response to the child. During these brief seconds, I concentrate on my breathing and being present in the moment. I then intentionally come back into the present moment with the child and work to offer feeling reflections to move into empathic understanding of the child's world. Therapist dysregulation in session is a symptom of permeable boundaries in which the therapist has allowed the child's world to become the therapist's world. Empathic understanding is marked by the therapist experiencing the world of the child while still knowing it is a separate world from their own.

Child dysregulation is an expected and frequent event in play therapy. Many of our child clients live in a dysregulated world and react accordingly. Dysregulation becomes part of their everyday response to their environment. In my experience, children become dysregulated when they are out of connection with others, and their behaviors become more disturbing during these periods of disconnection. Therefore, I seek to come into relational connection with children who are dysregulated. I will attempt to make eye contact with a child as my first response. Secondly, I will move in closer proximity to the child in a nonthreatening, slow manner, just to let them know I am here with them. I will intentionally slow down my breathing and may do so audibly to model for the child. I will soften my voice and make feeling reflections to let the child know I am trying to understand them. If the child does not feel threatened, I will sometimes reach out to touch the child on the shoulder or back. Soft and safe touch is often reassuring to a child who is dysregulated. In all times of dysregulation, I work to send a message of safety to the child that I am a safe person and the child is in a safe place. The child's process of moving from dysregulation to regulation is a crucial part of developing effective coping skills for dealing with adversity.

Jessica Stone, PhD, RPT-S

Regulation and dysregulation both have a place in play therapy work. Both states provide valuable windows into one's experience, perspective, concerns, and worldview. How a person moves between and within these states can help identify areas of needed intervention. Where do these states happen? What are the triggers? What skills work and which do not?

Emotional regulation is at the base of one's ability to function within their culture and society. The ability to manage emotional responses and understand how such internal experiences can drive behaviors equates to different forms of success within society. The question for me is less "What is the importance of regulation in my play therapy work" and more "What is the importance of regulation in my client's life/experience?"

The measurement of regulation and dysregulation states can be obvious with clear adherence to social norms (regulation) or big, overt, socially challenging behaviors (dysregulation). However, these states can also manifest in less overt ways. They can contribute to a more internalized process where the client is experiencing calm or distress without obvious external exhibition. Whether the display is overt or internal, the effect of a repeated experience of dysregulation can be exponential and effect self-esteem, relationships, social skills, and more. It is important to conceptualize this as a continuum with regulation and dysregulation on the left and right end of an axis and long term and short-term effects on the upper and lower ends of an axis (Figure 9.1).

Instances of dysregulation are often reported either by the client through sharing experiences from different environments such as school, home, after-school activities, and social situations or via the adults in his/her life through communications, written reports, or behavioral consequences. One important aspect of these experiences is to explore any identifiable triggers such as verbal, nonverbal, tactile, visceral, smells, and sounds, whether they occur in or out of session. Helping the client understand what leads to their states of dysregulation can assist them in thwarting the occurrences or, at a minimum, reducing the impact of them.

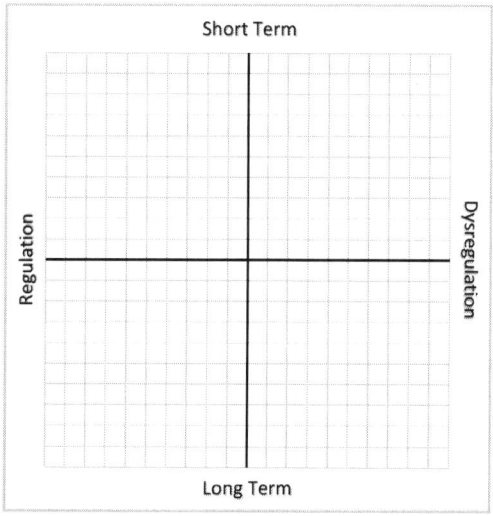

Figure 9.1 Continuum of Regulation and Dysregulation: Short and Long Term.

Daniel Sweeney, PhD, RPT-S

I am most interested in emotional regulation – really *coregulation* – more than I am in other areas of regulation. Schore (2010) asserts, "Secure attachment depends not on the mother's psychobiological attunement with the infant's cognition or behavior, but rather on her regulation of the infant's internal states of arousal, the energetic dimension of the child's affective state" (p. 20). He also states that coregulation involves a caregiver accurately "reading" the infant's nonverbal affective communications and adjusting his or her somato-sensory signals to restore equilibrium (Schore, 1994). I want to promote this in the playroom and in the parent training process.

Patton and Benedict (2014) contend that in play therapy

> the therapist needs to act as a coregulator of the child's emotions and be-havior because traumatized children have difficulties with self-regulation. This is done in various ways, including reflecting feelings and helping children know how the therapist recognizes their feelings so that they can thereby know their own feelings
>
> (p. 24)

This is a key element to establishing regulation. This is also a key teaching and modeling part of the filial therapy process (Landreth & Bratton, 2020). Children also experience regulation through hearing and responding limits in the play therapy process (Landreth, 2012; Landreth & Bratton, 2020).

Perry (2006) asserts that for traumatized children, normal brain development is fundamentally interrupted, which causes problems with emotional regulation, thus further interrupting children's ability to think, communicate, and relate. This, in turn, points to the key issue of relationship – in play therapy and in the family environment. Regulation is best established within the context of safe relationships. Perry and Pate (1994) emphasize this point:

> It is the 'relationship' which enables access to parts of the brain involved in social affiliation, attachment, arousal, affect, anxiety regulation and physiological hyper-reactivity. Therefore, the elements of therapy which induce positive changes will be the relationship and the ability of the child to re-experience traumatic events in the context of a safe and supportive relationship. (p. 142)

References

Badenoch, B. (2008). *Being a brain-wise therapist: A practical guide to interpersonal neurobiology*. Norton.

Blaustein, M. E., & Kinniburgh, K. (2010). *Treating traumatic stress in children and adolescents: How to foster resilience through attachment, self-regulation, and competency*. The Guilford Press.Eisenberg, N., Hofer, C., & Vaughan, J. (2007). Effortful control and its socioemotional consequences. In J. J. Gross (Ed.), *Handbook of emotion regulation* (pp. 287–306). Guilford.

Eisenberg, N., & Sulik, M. J. (2012). Emotion-related self-regulation in children. *Teaching of Psychology, 39*, 77–83.

Eisenberg, N. Spinrad, T. L., & Eggum, N. D. (2010). Emotion-related self-regulation and its relation to children's maladjustment. *Annual Review of Clinical Psychology, 6*, 496–525.

Goodyear-Brown, P. (2010). *Play therapy with traumatized children: A prescriptive approach*. Wiley.

Hebert, M., Langevin, R., & Oussaid, E. (2018). Cumulative childhood trauma, emotion regulation, dissociation, and behavior problems in school-aged sexual abuse victims. *Journal of Affective Disorders, 225*, 306–312.

Kaduson, H. G. (2015). Release play therapy for children with posttraumatic stress disorder. In H. G. Kaduson & C. E. Schaefer (Eds.), *Short-term play therapy for children* (3rd ed., pp. 3–24). Guilford Press.

Knell, S. M. (1993). To show and not tell: Cognitive-behavioral play therapy. In T. Kottman & C. E. Schaefer (Eds.), *Play therapy in action: A casebook for practitioners*. Jason Aronson.

Landreth, G. (2012). *Play therapy: The art of the relationship* (3rd ed.). Routledge.

Landreth, G., & Bratton, S. (2020). *Child-parent relationship therapy (CPRT): An evidence-based 10-session filial therapy model* (2nd ed.). Routledge.

Ogden, P., & Minton, K. (2000). Sensorimotor psychotherapy: One method for processing traumatic memory. *Traumatology, 6*(3), 149–173. doi:10.1177/153476560000600302Patton, S., & Benedict, H. (2014). Object relations and attachment-based play therapy. In D. Crenshaw & A. Stewart (Eds.), *Play therapy: A comprehensive guide to theory and practice* (pp. 3–16). Guilford Publications.

Perry, B. (2006). Applying principles of neurodevelopment to clinical work with maltreated and traumatized children. In N. B. Webb (Ed.), *Working with traumatized youth in child welfare* (pp. 27–52). Guilford Press.

Perry, B., & Pate, J. (1994). Neurodevelopment and the psychobiological roots of post-traumatic stress disorder. In L. Koziol & C. Stout (Eds.), *The neuropsychology of mental disorders: A practical guide* (pp. 129–146). Charles C. Thomas Publisher.

Perry, B., & Szalavitz, M. (2006). *The boy who was raised as a dog: What traumatized children teach us about loss, love and healing.* Basic Books.

Sbarra, D. A., & Hazan, C. (2008). Coregulation, dysregulation, self-regulation: An integrative analysis and empirical agenda for understanding adult attachment, separation, loss and recovery. *Personality and Social Psychology Review, 12*, 141–167.

Schore, A. (1994). *Affect regulation and the origin of the self: The neurobiology of emotional development.* Erlbaum.

Schore, A. (2010). Relational trauma and the developing right brain: The neurobiology of broken attachment bonds. In T. Baradon (Ed.), *Relational trauma in infancy* (pp. 19– 47). Routledge.

Siegel, D. J. (1999). *The developing mind: Toward a neurobiology of interpersonal experience.* Guilford Press.

Siegal, D. J. (2012). *The developing mind: How relationship and the brain interact to shape who we are* (2nd ed.). Guilford Press.

van der Kolk, B. A. (2014). *The body keeps the score: Brain, mind, and body in the healing of trauma.* Viking.

Vygotsky, L. S. (1978). *Mind in society: The development of higher psychological processes.* Harvard University Press.

Warner, E., Cook, A., Westcott, A., & Koomar, J. (2011). Sensory motor arousal regulation treatment (SMART), a manual for therapists working with children and adolescents: A "bottom-up" approach to treatment of complex trauma. Trauma Center at JRI.

10 How Do You Incorporate Nature into Play Therapy Treatment?

Jeff Ashby, PhD, RPT-S

While I am personally very connected to nature, it is not a direct component of my play therapy work. However, the eclecticism of technique that is a hallmark of AdPT does include interventions that incorporate nature. For instance, with selected clients, I might use techniques of Adventure Therapy (Ashby et al., in press), the use of a sequence of active games, activities, challenges, and trust exercises designed to promote desired therapeutic outcomes for clients. While not a requirement, Adventure Therapy traditionally incorporates various aspects of nature and is often conducted outside (Martin & Ashby, 2008). In my practice of Adventure Therapy techniques, I regularly take clients (especially in groups) outside and incorporate nature into the treatment.

While the incorporation of nature is not a direct component of AdPT, connection to the natural world is an important aspect of the goals of therapy. One of the primary goals of AdPT is the promotion of social interest, the sense of connectedness with self, others, and the planet (Kottman & Meany-Walen, 2016). This sense of connectedness to the planet can be fostered through overt interventions that incorporate nature (e.g., adventure therapy) or be developed in conjunction with interventions designed to foster connectedness to self and others.

Robert Jason Grant, EdD, RPT-S

Nature can be a powerful and effective modality in working with children in play therapy. It provides the opportunity to explore play in ways that might not be manifested in a traditional play therapy setting. Research is growing and showing support for using nature and nature-based interventions in working with children in play therapy (Swank & Smith-Adcock, 2018).

I have practiced in four play therapy mental health settings in my career. One of the settings I worked in had a large private sensory playground which included grass, trees, bushes, and a garden. During my time in this setting, I would spend many sessions in the playground with clients and most of this time was child-led. Many children preferred to be outside even just to sit in a swing and talk. I think nature holds a great appeal to children. For many clients there is a grounding affect. I witnessed this often while I worked in the clinic with the sensory playground. That setting communicated clearly to me how important nature can be in the play therapy process.

When I moved from the sensory playground clinic to my current clinic space, I found myself back in a situation with no opportunity to be outdoors. What I learned from the sensory playground was the importance and value of nature in play therapy. The goal for me has been to find ways to include nature in my current work which does not support being outside. Langley (2019) described several ways by which nature can be brought indoors including having a variety of nature objects in a wooden bowl or basket that the child can take out and touch, feel, and smell. Leaves can be very calming, just by having the child trace with his or her fingers along the veins of the leaf. Pebbles and rocks can be held for calming due to the grounding nature of the stones. Children can use various nature objects and place them in patterns and formations as another way to provide regulation in a playful yet intentional manner.

I have incorporated these ideas and several others. Being in a setting that does not have an outdoor space, I have had to become more mindful of how to include nature inside my playroom. Additional ideas I have implemented include having children create a nature mandala (gather the materials and have them available in your playroom), having a nature-based (leaves, acorns, grass seed) sand tray available for children to use, having water trays in the playroom, a variety of rocks for writing or painting affirmations on, or as a transition item children can take home when their session is over. I have also begun to include live plants and herbs growing in my playroom space. There are several ideas that can bring nature more into the playroom. It requires a bit of exploration and thoughtfulness, but I have found it to be very worthwhile.

Heidi Gerard Kaduson, PhD, RPT-S

Nature is part of play therapy because it is in all of us. There are some children who need to do their play outside with the grass, trees, or water, and there are others that use the sand tray or set up what they perceive nature to be for themselves. If the child is from an inner city, the needs could be different than a child from the country. I follow the child's lead but am always open to incorporating some part of nature. A typical process I have noticed is for a child to create a nature scene to play out on the floor of the playroom, and they utilize nature elements in the creation. Whenever possible, I suggest we add some nature pieces from outside. We go outside, and the child collects acorns, pine-cones, sticks and stones, whatever they like. They come back and seem to know exactly what they want to do and where each item will be placed. Often the smell of nature seems to help children to release tension and work through even difficult traumatic events. I have also found that for some children – in order to play their own way – they request to do things outside (which is accomplished if the weather permits). Their connection with nature and play is innate, and it is easy to join them and follow.

Jennifer Lefebre, PsyD, RPT-S

I am blessed that my current practice is located on a river. I often go outside with my clients to sit on the bench on the back patio that overlooks the river, and there has been a peacefulness to throwing rocks into the river. Setting up yoga mats on the grass to incorporate trauma-sensitive yoga adds a peaceful-ness not found inside, and drumming outdoors creates beautiful rhythms with nature. This area also allows for the finding of sticks, many stones, flowers, and leaves to incorporate into all elements of play therapy. I have been fed a mud pie, have created nature mandalas, have planted flowers and a garden – and have many items being utilized within sand tray as well.

In general, I use many earth elements as metaphors, my favorites being trees and the ocean (which I use for self-care by creating mandalas in the sand tray). Metaphors involving weather seem to be particularly useful for understand-ing emotions. Grounding and calming strategies often come from nature, and most of my client's calm/peaceful places involve aspects of nature. Often, I will invite families to go on a nature walk together during the week between ses-sions. I ask them to practice the 5–4–3–2–1 exercise (author unknown) while they are on their walk to discover together: five things they can see, four things they can hear, three things they can feel, two things they can smell, and one thing they can taste, and compare and contrast their findings.

I am learning more about nature play therapy and I can't wait to incorporate it even more in my practice. I am finding the adults I work with are gravitating toward nature in so many ways, and I want to be able to incorporate nature play therapy even more into my practice.

Clair Mellenthin, MSW, RPT-S

"Involving nature in the therapeutic process brings out an innate drive to roam free, interact, make sense of, and explore the environment" (Hudspeth & Matthews, 2016, p. 595). I love to include nature in various capacities in my play therapy treatment. On my shelf of miniatures, there are items from nature that I have brought into the playroom such as rocks, seashells, twigs, sticks, geodes, feathers, and coral. I feel it is very important to have items related to both the local geography as well as other environments for use in the sand tray and for a child's therapeutic process.

My office is located in a neighborhood in a suburban area of a large city. It is located close to an elementary school with a large playground at the base of a large mountain range. I am lucky to live and work in a setting where nature is literally all around us and is a natural extension of the playroom. It is not uncommon to go for a nature walk and collect items of interest for use in play therapy with the child or family client. For children who need a break from big feelings or as a way to help regulate and calm down, we may take a "cool down" walk around the neighborhood or go to the park and use the swings. For children who need to "wake up" and rev up their internal emotional state, playing catch, hopscotch, and jumping or running games can be just what they need in the fresh air and sunshine to become focused and engaged. I always seek out parental permission before leaving the building premises, and when appropriate, invite the parents to come and engage in the therapeutic process.

I have used nature in various formats in play therapy. We have collected leaves from around the building to create a family mandala, created monster potions and spells using "ingredients" from outside (smashed dead bugs are great for this!), and have built fairy habitats out of sticks and grass. I love to use nature-only items in sand tray work, where the client collects items of interest from the outdoors and then uses these instead of the commercial store-bought miniatures to process their world, their thoughts and feelings, and how they see themselves and their relationships. This can be an incredibly powerful way to utilize nature in sand tray work. This is also, by far, one of my favorite interventions to use when I am facilitating a sand tray workshop – especially when we can use a beach as the sand tray!

Akiko J. Ohnogi, PsyD

I am in support of nature being incorporated into play therapy treatment if the clinician is comfortable with and knows how to utilize nature therapeutically. There are many aspects of the natural world that can positively stimulate and have an effect on a person's senses and unconscious thoughts and feelings (Mygind et al., 2019). If one were incorporating exposure interventions for post-trauma work related to a nature-based trauma (floods, hurricane, earthquake, etc.), then the utilization of nature can be quite powerful in healing the brain. This is because nature-based interventions will access the unconscious, sensory, and emotional areas of the brain where the trauma memories reside, and have an immediate effect (Song et al., 2016). Because it is so powerful, caution must be taken when doing this, and the play therapist must be comfortable with and well-trained in what they are doing, otherwise the danger of retraumatizing the client can be extensive.

I wish I had an office or natural setting to utilize for treatment. Unfortunately, I am located in mid-center Tokyo and lack access to private areas within nature that would provide appropriate confidentiality. I have attended quite a few workshops throughout the years on nature-based play therapy, but due to lack of practicality, I have not been able to incorporate most of what has been suggested. Instead, in my playroom I have many plants and fresh flowers, have nature objects to use (e.g., rocks, leaves, shells), play music with nature sounds, and use nature-inspired imagery techniques.

Mary Anne Peabody, EdD, RPT-S

Interestingly, while I have nature items (leaves, rocks, sticks) in my sand tray materials, I rarely bring clients outside in my private practice. However, as a school-based play therapist, I often bring my play therapy clients into the school playground or surrounding nature walks. We would occasionally go on "walk and talks" (Doucette, 2004) or have conversations as we swing on the playground structures. In school-based group play therapy, the playground is often used as our "real life" learning laboratory and a natural setting to promote social skill development.

Peter Gray (2011) has voiced concerns over the lack of outside play for children and adolescents. There are many compounding challenges that contribute to the changing landscape of play for children (Brown & Vaughn, 2009; Yogman et al., 2018) and as play therapists I believe helping parents, children, and teachers find a balance in activities is part of our responsibility. Living life with a balanced equation of time inside and outside, providing both structured and unstructured play activities all contribute to overall social, emotional, and physical well-being (Yogman et al., 2018).

I am curious about the growing scholarship in nature-based play therapy (Courtney & Mills, 2016; Swank & Shin, 2015; Swank et al., 2017) and wonder how play therapists will explore this arena of practice. I can see this as an area of ongoing learning for myself, as I fortunately practice in a beautiful nature-rich area where forests, ocean, and mountains are easily within reach. I personally experience a sense of wellness from simply being outside. Reflecting on this knowledge to enhance my own self-care only strengthens my ability to help others.

Dee Ray, PhD, RPT-S

In child-centered play therapy, I have stayed within the traditional provision of materials in a playroom (Landreth, 2012). However, I am a strong advocate for integrating nature into play therapy. I have been especially interested in Swank and Shin's (Swank & Shin, 2015; Swank et al., 2015) work on nature-based child-centered play therapy in which they have experimented with outdoor play sessions. In their work, they have developed cutting-edge modifications to child-centered protocol in order to provide children with the experience of a self-directed play approach in the context of the outdoors. Children are often innately drawn to the outdoors and the organic materials found there. There is a sense of freedom and awe experienced by children in nature which is a match with the principles of child-centered play therapy. Outdoor play sessions, when facilitated by child-centered play therapists, provide children an environment where they can experience themselves as capable in the greater world and bring them into connection with the world around them.

Jessica Stone, PhD, RPT-S

Luckily, my office has a good-sized backyard and tall fence that was purposely built for confidentiality reasons. This allows clients to utilize the backyard during sessions without the worry of being seen by the neighbors or from the street. A conversation about confidentiality with the client and parent/care-giver is important so that all parties can consider the possible ramifications of being outside the office with the therapist.

Working outside can include walking, talking, exploring, gathering, and playing. The backyard to my office has numerous trees, including a large one for shade, neighborhood cats, flowers, grass, dirt, bugs, and a detached garage. It is very common for sticks to become a number of items, such as wands, swords, fencing foils, canes, and more. Children often run and roll in the grass and climb into a low, flat portion of the large tree.

The incorporation of nature is primarily to provide an environment, and tools within such, for the client to express and experience what is desired and/or needed for them in the moment. There are times when even the sensation of a cool breeze on one's face can remind of a memory, energize, or even bring about an emotional response. Playing with sticks or other gathered materials can elicit interactions and responses in ways very similar to those found when playing inside: frustration tolerance, coping skills and styles, strategic abilities, interactional and intra-actional styles and skills, and so on (Stone, 2016).

Items can be gathered to contribute to art projects such as the "Me Doll" (Stone, 1997). As described in the book *101 Play Therapy Techniques*, the Me Doll involves tracing the child on large pieces of butcher paper and cutting out the tracing. This yields two identical cutouts which can be decorated with art materials on the outside and then stapled and stuffed with nature items identi-fied within the therapy to signify experiences, feelings, and/or characteristics. The Me Doll can be life-sized or a miniature version of the client or any other identified person.

It is also possible to find large outdoor versions of certain structured games such as Connect 4. There can be great fun in the management of the game when each game piece is approximately the size of a child's head. The game play can yield desired interactions and information, and the large components of the game offer novelty. It is also possible to play games such as mancala with stick and stones outdoors.

The connection to nature for some allows for a heightened level of safety and openness which is important to respect and cultivate. As with any iden-tified interest and safe environment, the play therapist would serve the client best by providing elements to the best of their ability. Identifying areas of interest, safety, and identification honors who the client is and their needs.

Daniel Sweeney, PhD, RPT-S

Nature is incorporated into my play therapy primarily through the materials provided in my playroom. These include such items as sand, dirt, feathers, seashells, driftwood, sticks, and leaves. Taking a primarily CCPT approach with young children I do not generally direct children to these items. With older children and adolescents, I may provide a directed activity with "natu-ral" items, if this seems appropriate. Most often, my work with nature in play therapy is within the context of sand tray therapy, where I have many more items that represent nature or come directly from nature.

I am intrigued with nature-based play therapy, discussed by Swank, Cheung, Prikhidko, and Su (2017). Their case was reminiscent of clinical work I did with group home preadolescents and adolescents when doing outdoor group activities. However, I would probably fit this under the category of therapeutic play rather than play therapy.

By and large, my play therapy is limited to work in the play therapy room. I see significant potential with outdoor therapeutic activities, but issues related to environmental constraints and confidentiality make this an approach where I am limited.

References

Ashby, J. S., Jin, M. K., & Tobin, G. (2020). Adlerian play therapy and adventure therapy: Complimentary interventions for a comprehensive theory. *Journal of Individual Psychology*, 76:187–200.

Brown, S., & Vaughn, C. (2009). *Play: How it shapes the brain, opens the imagination, and invigorates the soul.* Penguin Group.

Courtney, J. A., & Mills, J. C. (2016). Utilizing the metaphor of nature as co-therapist in StoryPlay®. *Play Therapy*, 11(1), 18–21.

Doucette, P. A. (2004). Walk and talk: An intervention for behaviorally challenged youth. *Adolescence*, 39(154), 373–388.

Gray, P. (2011). The decline of play and the rise of psychopathology in children and adolescents. *American Journal of Play*, 3(4), 443–463.

Hudspeth, E. F., & Matthews, K. (2016). Neuroscience and play therapy: The neurobiologically informed play therapist. In K. J. O'Connor, C. E. Schaefer, & L. D. Braverman (Eds.), *Handbook of play therapy* (2nd ed., pp. 583–598). Wiley.

Kottman, T., & Meany-Walen, K. (2016). *Partners in play: An Adlerian approach to play therapy* (3rd ed.). American Counseling Association.

Landreth, G., (2012). *Play therapy: The art of the relationship* (3rd ed.). Routledge.

Langley, J. L. (2019). Nature play therapy: When nature comes into play. *Playground* (Spring/Summer), 20–24. https://cacpt.com/wpcontent/uploads/2019/04/Playground-Spring-2019.pdf.

Martin, J. M., & Ashby, J. S. (2008). Adventure counseling. In F. Leong (Ed.), *Encyclopedia of Counseling* (pp. 12–14). Sage.

Mygind, L., Kjeldsted, E., Hartmeyer, R. D., Mygind, R., Bolling, M., & Bentsen, P. (2019). Immersive nature-experiences as health promotion interventions for healthy, vulnerable, and sick populations? A systematic review and appraisal of controlled studies. *Frontiers in Psychology*. https://doi.org/10.3389/fpsyg.2019.00943.

Song, C., Ikei, H., & Miyazaki, Y. (2016). Physiological effects of nature therapy: A review of the research in Japan. *International Journal of Environmental Research and Public Health*. https://www.ncbi.nlm.nih.gov/pmc/articles/PMC4997467/.

Stone, J. (1997). The me doll. In H. G. Kaduson & C. E. Schaefer (Eds.), *101 play therapy techniques*. Aaronson.

Stone, J. (2016). Board game play therapy. In K. O'Connor, C. Schaefer, & L. Braverman (Eds.), *The handbook of play therapy* (2nd ed., pp. 309–323). Wiley.

Swank, J. M., Cheung, C., Prikhidko, A., & Su, Y. W. (2017). Nature-based child-centered group play therapy and behavioral concerns: A single-case design. *International Journal of Play Therapy, 26*(1), 47–57.

Swank, J. M., & Shin, S. M. (2015). Nature-based child-centered play therapy: An innovative counseling approach. *International Journal of Play Therapy, 24*(3), 151–161. doi:10.1037/a0039127.

Swank, J. M., Shin, S. M., Carita, C., Cheung, C., & Rivers, B. (2015). Initial investigation of nature-based, child-centered play therapy: A single-case design. *Journal of Counseling & Development, 93*, 440–450. doi:10.1002/jcad.12042.

Swank, J. M., & Smith-Adcock, S. (2018). On-task behavior of children with attention deficit/hyperactivity disorder: Examining treatment effectiveness of play therapy interventions. *International Journal of Play Therapy, 27*(4), 187–197.

Yogman, M., Garner, A., Hutchinson J., Hirsh-Pasek, K., Golinkoff, R. M. (2018). AAP Committee on psychosocial aspects of child and family health, AAP Council on communications and media. The power of play: A pediatric role in enhancing development in young children. *Pediatrics, 142*(3), 1–17.

11 How Do You Address Issues of Noncompliance and Aggression in the Playroom?

Jeff Ashby, PhD, RPT-S

In addressing issues of noncompliance and aggression in the playroom, I regularly look to the goal of the behavior. One of the primary principles of Adlerian psychology is that all behavior is goal directed (Ansbacher & Ansbacher, 1956). In trying to understand and alter the goals of children, I am reminded that "all misbehavior … stems from discouragement. The child lacks courage to behave in an active, constructive manner. A child does not misbehave unless he or she feels a real or threatened loss of status" (Dinkmeyer et al., 2007, pp. 11–12). Adlerian psychology suggests that the goals of discouraged children fall into four primary categories of striving: attention, power, revenge, and proving inadequacy (Dreikurs & Soltz, 1964). It is important for me to identify the goal of the behavior so that I can develop intervention strategies to fit the goal.

The practicalities of addressing issues of noncompliance and aggression in the playroom are acted on through limit-setting. Limit-setting is an important component of my play therapy practice because I strive to make therapy a cooperative experience that ultimately enhances clients' self-control and enhances their ability to consider alternate behavioral patterns. Consistent with the perspective of AdPT (e.g., Kottman & Meany-Walen, 2016), I try to limit behavior in anticipation of an act (while the client is clearly contemplating or preparing for inappropriate aggression or noncompliance) and engage in a four-step process. These steps are (1) stating the limit, (2) reflecting the child's feeling or metacommunicating about the underlying purpose of the aggression or noncompliance, (3) engaging the client in generating acceptable alternatives to the aggression or noncompliance, and (4) collaborating with the client to determine logical consequences if the client continues to break a limit.

Because I strive to develop an egalitarian relationship with the child (the first phase of therapy), I am doing my best to lay the groundwork for constructive limit-setting from the beginning of play therapy with a client. Even when using directive techniques with clients, I try to give choices and take care to share the power with the client. I am also fine with the expression of aggression in the playroom except in very limited settings (e.g., intentionally damaging toys, the playroom, themselves, or other clients). By reflecting clients' feelings and metacommunicating (the second step in the AdPT limit-setting process), working with the client to generate alternatives to the limit-breaking behavior (the third step), and agreeing on logical consequences (the fourth step), I am trying to help clients develop a sense of responsibility and self-efficacy, "using limit setting for the forces of good" (Kottman & Meany-Walen, 2016, p. 148).

Robert Jason Grant, EdD, RPT-S

Behavior is communication and the child who is being noncompliant or aggressive is communicating something. The key is to help the child with what is creating the behavior instead of focusing on the behavior and trying to force the child to stop the behavior. Noncompliant and aggressive behavior can have many "looks" and thus many reasons it is happening. Because of this, my approach would vary based on my understating of the child and what I believe the behavior is communicating. For me, there is not just one approach to addressing noncompliant or aggressive behavior and one of those approaches may be to do nothing depending on the context of what is happening.

One of the primary reasons I see noncompliant behavior is due to dysregulation. Many of the children I work with who have developmental disorders can easily become dysregulated. This dysregulation often leads to some form of noncompliant and/or aggressive behavior. The behavior is communicating that the child does not feel comfortable, does not feel safe, does not feel in control, and does not know what to do. In these situations, I would want to address the issue of dysregulation. I have worked with many children who begin the therapy process dysregulated. The environment is new, I am a new person, and this unfamiliarity can be very dysregulating. These children might not come out from under a chair in the lobby when they first come to therapy, or they may run up and down the hallways, or run out of the playroom, or display a variety of noncompliant behaviors.

One method I have implemented that has greatly reduced this dysregulation behavior is creating a social story about going to see a play therapist. I send the social story to the parents and ask them to read the story to their child several times before their first appointment. In the social story I discuss what the child will experience when they come to play therapy and there are pictures of the building, my playroom, and myself. This helps the child feel more familiar and comfortable when they come for their first session. My sample social story can be found on the AutPlay Therapy website (www.autplaytherapy.com). It should be noted that relationship development is crucial for helping alleviate many unwanted behaviors in the playroom. This should be the primary focus as therapy begins and continue to be present throughout therapy regardless of the therapeutic approach being implemented. Much behavior can likely be eliminated through solidly implemented relationship development.

I also utilize limit setting models when needed. If a behavior is to the point of needing to set a limit, I will typically utilize one of the limit setting models found in play therapy theory such as AutPlay Therapy (Grant, 2017), Child Centered Play Therapy (Landreth, 1991), Adlerian Play Therapy (Kottman & Meany-Walen, 2016), or Filial Therapy (VanFleet, 2014). I try to keep limit setting to a minimum. I prefer to focus on what the behavior is communicating and trying to address that communication. This is a big topic and so much of what a play therapist would do depends on knowing the child, what the child is doing, and the context in which the behavior is happening. I think therapists should certainly be mindful of behavior challenges, researching strategies, and feel comfortable in how they will address these issues when they present.

Heidi Gerard Kaduson, PhD, RPT-S

I use humor for both. I have never had a child aggressively go after me, but I will join a child's aggressive feelings and we both can fight off the bad guys or puppets or dinosaurs. I encourage the expression of aggression in the playroom. Since noncompliance can come from many different sources, I can generally say that if I sense that it is anxiety driven, I will do something very silly to break through it so that laughter begins. In most cases, the noncompliance is then gone. I am there to be a guide when needed, and a playful therapist at all times. I believe noncompliance comes from a mindset that is scared and afraid of what will come out in a therapist's office. What will the child feel after he or she says something about mom or dad? Will they feel they betrayed family members? Even in severe physical abuse cases, children do not start playing aggressively – they hold back and protect their family. I often have to encourage them to use the splatz eggs. I take one of the splatz and throw it at a white board, saying something general that I hate. The child is given another splatz and told to do the same. Most children enjoy saying what they hate, and while they love to throw the eggs, they are nervous about what they say. I reassure them that nothing can be heard by parents in the waiting room, and we all feel better getting our anger out and gone. So whatever aggressive play they want to do, I will join it in some form or another as permitted by the child.

Jennifer Lefebre, PsyD, RPT-S

The only directives or boundaries I have within the play therapy room are that we are gentle with each other and gentle with the toys. These two statements seem to be an umbrella for most "rules" or boundaries that could be needed not only in the play therapy room but in many other arenas as well. I use the word "gentle" rather than "safe", as it can be a trigger if a child has not ever truly felt safety or kindness. In my experiences, "gentle" is a word that tends to be less triggering for clients.

When a child is engaging in aggression or noncompliance, I try to find and reflect the underlying need to their behavior (e.g., it really seems like you need to _____) and then offer them solutions to meet that need (e.g., here is something you can _____). If a child is engaging in aggression/noncompliance toward items, I may say, "It looks like your hands need to break things right now, here are some things that can be broken". If a child is engaging in aggression/noncompliance toward a parent, sibling, or myself, I would reaffirm that in the play therapy room we are gentle with one another. A statement for this might be, "Dr. Jenn is not for biting/licking, but here are some things that are".

Most issues of noncompliance within my practice seem to occur when ending the session or cleaning up, potentially originating from an undeveloped sense of object constancy, or the emotional equivalence of object permanence (Sherwood, 1989). As I work predominantly with children who have been through trauma and the corresponding disruptions in attachment, it makes sense that their ability to trust in the therapeutic relationship is challenged as they cannot always hold that their bonds with others remain whole even when they are not physically near. Developmental trauma leads to the belief that separation means disappearance or abandonment, so when a loved one is temporarily out of sight, they do not feel loved or supported. Play therapy activities that promote affectively attuned mirroring and object constancy (i.e., peekaboo, hide and seek, funhouse mirrors, yoga dance) support and grow the understanding that others continue to exist even when they cannot be seen, touched, or sensed in some way. In these cases, I will give the child additional time to transition out of the next session, and often focus on developing a ritual for leaving therapy, which may include a transitional item as deemed clinically appropriate. By following the child's lead, we can discover and meet the needs of the attachment seeking behavior which typically drives noncompliance.

Clair Mellenthin, MSW, RPT-S

I tend to use humor and relationship building to diffuse difficult situations where noncompliance is occurring in the playroom or more commonly in my experience, in the waiting room. I find if I don't get locked into a power struggle with my clients, typically these events tend to be fleeting. The child is attempting to communicate with me and it is my job to not get locked into "who is the boss" but to understand and empathize with the child that "yes, going into the playroom can be scary, overwhelming, intimidating", and I am another adult in their life who they may not want to work with in that moment. Often, underlying the defiance is a fear that I won't really like them if I see "the dark parts" of self. This is an attachment issue that needs nurture and consistency, as well as healthy boundaries in place. This can also be a good opportunity to model other, more appropriate parenting techniques for parents who are witnessing this interaction.

To address aggression in the playroom, I tend to follow Landreth's ACT limit setting and follow his sage advice, "Limits are not needed until they are needed" (2002, p. 248). The ACT limit setting protocol (Landreth, 2002) is as follows:

Step 1: Acknowledge the child's feelings, wishes, and wants.
Step 2: Communicate the limit.
Step 3: Target acceptable alternatives.

I feel that giving acceptable alternatives is an important aspect of limit setting. It is also important for the play therapist to remember that the child is trying to communicate something big and important with you, albeit through more maladaptive means. Often when a child has gone through overwhelming, big experiences they feel big emotions and they have big behaviors. When you appear to be intimidated or scared of the behaviors, the child may internalize that you are scared of them, which can create an attachment injury in the therapeutic relationship. It is important to remember that there is a difference between aggression and aggressive play. Both may need limit setting to provide for safety and containment, but it is so important to allow for aggressive play for both male and female children to work through their difficult emotions and experiences. If we stunt or limit all aggression-themed play, we may be limiting important parts of self that need to be explored and processed.

Akiko J. Ohnogi, Psy.D.

To address noncompliance and aggression in the play therapy room, I enforce limit setting in stages. I advocate the following six-step limit setting procedure (Ohnogi, 2013; 2019). At each step, I will communicate to the child and wait for the child's response before deciding whether to proceed to the next step. Steps 1 and 2 are sometimes combined, unless a specific behavior can be stopped by verbalizing the emotion without verbalizing the actual limit.

1   Reflect emotions and cause of emotion, "You are really mad at me because I won't leave the room for a few minutes".
2   State the limit, "You can't hit me with that bat".
3   Suggest an alternative behavior, "You can pretend that large stuffed alligator is me and hit it instead or make me out of playdoh and mash it".
4   State the consequence, "If you choose to try to hit me then you can't use the bat the rest of this session".
5   Implement the consequence, "Ok, you've chosen to try to hit me, so you've decided not to use the bat the rest of this session". I would take away the bat for the rest of the session, no matter how much the child cries, pleads, has tantrums, cozies up, and so on.

6   Reflect emotions and repeat the stated consequence, "You are upset that you can't use the bat anymore today because you chose to try to hit me. You can use it again next week if you want".

Oftentimes, when I reflect the child's emotion and state the rule, the child is able to follow through without having to continue with the next steps of limit setting. I have not had to address actual physical violence except with siblings becoming physically aggressive with one another. I would probably not intervene physically unless absolutely necessary,

My basic rule in the playroom is that the child does not have to do anything they do not want to do, except to not harm themselves, me, or the toys and furniture. They must end their play and leave the room when it is time. Thus, if the child chooses not to play, speak, respond, interact, engage, and so on, whether it be for unstructured play or structured activities, I will continue reflecting their feelings that accompany their behavior and do not consider it noncompliance.

Mary Anne Peabody, EdD, RPT-S

Aggression and noncompliance are not behaviors that my clients typically display during playroom sessions. Perhaps, it is the one-to-one experience or the type of children I typically work with, but if I need to set limits for noncompliance or aggression, I use the child-centered approach of limiting setting and choice giving as my strategies (Landreth, 2012). Having spent a significant number of years in elementary public schools as a therapist, I am also behaviorally trained in recognizing the role of the environment and antecedents to escalating behavior. This knowledge and skill set has fine-tuned my awareness of environmental cues, redirection, and the creative use of playfulness when working with children in the school or therapy setting.

In the rare occasions that aggression does enter the place and space of the playroom, I view this as a way to utilize one of the therapeutic powers of play, namely catharsis, and this typically involves physical release of some sort (Drewes & Schaefer, 2014). My training has included that cathartic experiences in the playroom should be paired with intentional cognitive and emotional processing support, such as the labeling the child's feelings out loud so that the physical release is designed for integration, reframing, or reeducation (Drewes & Schaefer, 2014). Children often used my foam pool noodles or sponge blocks for the releasing of physical energy.

I also spend time during parental consultation in psychoeducation regarding how behavior is a child's way of communicating unmet needs. I share that even as children mature, verbally communicating big feelings can still be a challenge and that our job is to figure out, interpret, and address the need underneath the behavior. This requires that we are regulated ourselves and able to approach the child with the intent and skill set to share our calm, not contribute to escalating the situation.

Dee Ray, PhD, RPT-S

In child-centered play therapy, aggressive and limit-breaking behaviors exhibited by children are attempts to fulfill their needs, an incongruence between the self and environment that manifests through problematic behaviors with others. By the time children who are aggressive reach play therapy, they have typically experienced the confusion between personal need and aggressive acts so many times that they have developed a rigid set of coping skills to meet their needs. "The great irony of effective child therapy is that the more children feel understood and accepted in their current rigid ways of meeting their needs, the more they feel free to explore alternative courses of action" (Ray, 2017, p. 192). Sending the message that the child is understood and that their needs are worthy of meeting is the foundation of working effectively with children who act aggressively. Thus, the process of working with children who are aggressive is communicating empathic understanding through reflections of feelings, needs, and desires.

I seek to send the message that I see what you are feeling or what you want and that feeling or want is important to me. The feeling or desire of the child is the most important factor in our interaction, even when limits of behavior are necessary. A highly effective method for sending this message while addressing problem behaviors is the use of ACT limit-setting technique (Landreth, 2012). The steps of ACT include acknowledging the child's feelings or desires (e.g., "you are angry …", "you want to be the one who decides …"), communicating the limit (e.g., "but I am not for hitting", "but the room is not for leaving"), and targeting an alternative (e.g., "you can hit the bop bag", "you can leave in 10 minutes"). With ACT, the therapist prioritizes the child's needs while setting the limit that certain behaviors are not acceptable. The child is **always** accepted even when the child's behaviors are not. Through ACT, the child is faced with the dissonance that what I want and feel is of worth but I need to find a new way to express this way-of-being to move toward self-enhancing behaviors.

What I truly love about using ACT is observing children as they move through the process of running up against a limit, confusion that the adult is not going to deny their needs, and the resulting experimental behaviors to develop new coping skills. For example, in working with a child who wants to leave the playroom, I may say, "You're wanting to leave the room but the room is not for leaving right now, you can leave in 10 minutes when our time is up". For children who are referred for aggressive behaviors, the child might respond with yelling, arguing, throwing toys, and even physical aggression. As I continue to calmly and supportively set the limit, the child tries old coping skills that have previously worked whereby the adult gives in, becomes dysregulated, or aggressively responds to the child. Once the child sees that the old coping skills no longer are effective, they start to engage in all new coping skills to get their needs met within appropriate behavioral boundaries. The process can be long and challenging for the child and the therapist but completely worth the struggle.

Jessica Stone, PhD, RPT-S

Long ago I worked in an endodontic office as a registered dental assistant. I learned many things while working in that environment and some important concepts have informed everything from the way I speak with clients and families, how I work with collateral contacts, and the awareness of the client's experience from the moment they arrive at the office. I would frequently sit in the dental chair and look around so I could see what the patient could see from their perspective. I would do my best to imagine what their experience with us might be. In a sense, I applied a prescriptive approach before I even knew what that was by altering the environment and my approach according to their needs. The environment sets the stage for the upcoming interactions.

I have been fortunate enough to purchase a small home for my office and renovate as desired. This allowed a good amount of latitude when designing the intended experience for the client from walking up to the door, sitting in the waiting room, and choosing a room in which to work that day. The experience is based in comfort, safety, and mutual respect. The space is congruent with who I am as a human and a psychologist and people reflect that the experience is positive.

All this is to say that the experience a client has starts before they even walk in the door, continues with the "feel" of the environment, and builds with the relationship between the client and therapist. When a client is "noncompliant" or "aggressive" in the playroom, which rarely happens in my practice, it is important for the therapist to work to understand what is underneath the behaviors. Addressing those components typically results in the cessation of the behaviors, at a minimum in the office, with the goal of integrating such self-regulating tools and understandings into day-to-day life outside of the office.

Limit setting is an important personal and professional journey for a play therapist. It is imperative that a therapist understand what limits should be in place and why; which are about the therapist and which are about the client; which are about safety and which are about clinical messages; and so on. These are predominately tailored to the therapist, the underlying theoretical foundation, and the therapeutic approach. Once the environment is safe, connection is a fundamental goal. The therapist must listen, *really listen to hear*, and cue in to the verbal and nonverbal communications. Human beings want to feel heard, seen, understood, and accepted. When this is accomplished the noncompliance and aggression is either greatly reduced or extinguished.

Daniel Sweeney, PhD, RPT-S

Children are frequently referred for issues of noncompliance and aggression. These are particularly challenging for parents and teachers. However, they should be routinely expected for the play therapist.

Before addressing dealing with these issues, I would like to comment on aggression in general. The Gestalt perspective on aggression is helpful to remember:

> Aggression serves the life of the child and allows distinctions to be made between the child and the environment. The child's ability to regress allows the two-year old to become more independent, while remaining embedded within the support of the family. Aggression mobilizes the young child to reach out and make new friends, or ask for what she wants. From the Gestalt view, aggression enables the child to orient, mobilize, and organize her excitement or energy. Aggression, therefore, is essential for contact. It is life itself.
>
> (Carroll, 2009, p. 285)

Aggression may be a call for help from the child, or it may be a way to protect the self from a dangerous world. It is not negative in and of itself. It can obviously, however, be harmful and thus needs to be addressed.

Children should be allowed to express aggression in the playroom. This may be challenging for some play therapists, who may too quickly set limits on aggressive behavior. However, if a child is not able to express aggression in the controlled yet relational setting of play therapy, where else can this be explored?

Children should not be allowed to aggress toward self, the therapist, or other children when physical or emotional safety may be compromised. Additionally, aggressive expressions which involve breaking playroom materials simply to break them is not acceptable. There should be, however, play materials that are purposefully provided with which to express aggression and to break. Also, although the philosophy behind this is beyond the scope of this short chapter, I personally endorse the provision of aggressive toys in the playroom, including toy dart guns and inflatable bop bags. When children are expressing anger and aggression, they can be given acceptable means to express these behaviors and emotions, through aggressive toys [see Crenshaw (2015), Kottman and Meany-Walen (2016), and Landreth (2012)].

I use Landreth's (2012) therapeutic limit setting model with aggression. At the same time, I do not set limits on noncompliance in the play room – it is not my position that any behavior in the playroom is "noncompliant" – unless it is expressed in the form of inappropriate aggression. Additionally, I teach this therapeutic limit setting model to parents in the filial therapy (Landreth & Bratton, 2020) parent training process.

References

Ansbacher, H., & Ansbacher, R. (Eds.). (1956). *The individual psychology of Alfred Adler: A systematic presentation in selections from his writings.* Harper and Row.

Carroll, F. (2009). Gestalt play therapy. In K. O'Connor & L. Braverman (Eds.), *Play therapy and practice: Comparing theories and techniques* (2nd ed., pp. 283–314). John Wiley & Sons.

Crenshaw, D. (2015). Play therapy with "children of fury": Treating the trauma of betrayal. In D. Crenshaw & A. Stewart (Eds.), *Play therapy: A comprehensive guide to theory and practice* (pp. 217–231). Guilford Publications.

Dinkmeyer, D., McKay, G., & Dinkmeyuer, D. (2007). *The parent's handbook: Systematic Training for Effective Parenting (STEP)* (Rev. ed.). American Guidance Service.

Dreikurs, R., & Soltz, V. (1964). *Children: The challenge.* Hawthorn/Dutton.

Drewes, A. A., & Schaefer, C. E. (2014). Catharsis. In C. E. Schaefer & A. A. Drewes (Eds.), *The therapeutic powers of play: Twenty core agents of change* (2nd ed., pp. 71–81). Wiley.

Grant, R. J. (2017). *AutPlay therapy for children and adolescents on the autism spectrum: A behavioral play-based approach.* Routledge.

Kottman, T., & Meany-Walen, K. (2016). *Partners in play: An Adlerian approach to play therapy* (3rd ed.). American Counseling Association.

Landreth, G. L. (1991). *Play therapy: The art of the relationship.* Accelerated Development Inc. Publishers.

Landreth, G. L. (2002). *Play therapy: The art of the relationship* (2nd ed.). Brunner-Routledge.

Landreth, G. L. (2012). *Play therapy: The art of the relationship* (3rd ed.). Brunner-Routledge.

Landreth, G., & Bratton, S. (2020). *Child-parent relationship therapy (CPRT): An evidence-based 10-session filial therapy model* (2nd ed.). Routledge.

Ohnogi, A. (2013). Creating a psychologically safe and accepting space through limit setting in play therapy. *International Journal of Counseling and Psychotherapy, 10–11,* 75–80.

Ohnogi, A. (2019). *My first play therapy: Basics and techniques for effective support.* Seishin Shobo (In Japanese only. *Hajimete no Purei Serapi – Koukateki na Shien no tame no Kiso to Gihou*).

Ray, D. (2017). Relating when relating is hard: Working with aggression in play therapy. In S. Daniel & C. Trevarthen (Eds.), *Rhythms of relating in children's therapies* (pp. 188–206). Jessica Kingsley.

Sherwood, V. R. (1989). Object constancy: The illusion of being seen. *Psychoanalytic Psychology,* 6(1), 15–30. doi:10.1037/0736-9735.6.1.15.

VanFleet, R. (2014). *Filial therapy: Strengthening parent-child relationships through play* (3rd ed.). Professional Resource Press.

12 How Do You Use a Sand Tray in Your Play Therapy Work?

Jeff Ashby, PhD, RPT-S

As indicated earlier, the eclecticism of technique in AdPT allows me to use a sand tray in each phase of therapy. The value of sand tray work is that it allows me to access a child's unconscious thoughts and feelings and can give a clear visual depiction of the child's inner world. Depending on the phase of treatment and the lifestyle and preferences of the client, I may use a sand tray in any number of ways. One advantage of using a sand tray is, as Carey (1990) notes, "Sand is tactile, yet provides a total kinesthetic involvement. This leads to a concentrated focus or meditative space that allows the inner, protected self to emerge" (p. 198). I believe that sand tray work can provide clients a safe way to deal with painful experiences or personal struggles in a nonthreatening and sometimes unconscious way and can be used all phases of therapy.

I tend to use sand tray work early in the first phase of therapy to learn about the client and assess the client's interest and enthusiasm for the medium. Some clients are naturally drawn to the sand and, as a result, I am more likely to utilize it as a medium for intervention and assessment later in the therapy. Both structured and unstructured trays can be an effective means of collecting information about the client's lifestyle. Especially in early trays, I note any representation of family dynamics, functioning at life tasks, mistaken beliefs, and other lifestyle components (Bainum et al., 2006). In the third phase of therapy (helping the child gain insight into lifestyle), I may use directed trays designed to help the client gain insight. In similar fashion, I may construct a tray for the client or cocreate trays with clients as a means of giving a client feedback about their lifestyle. An example might be a tray where the client and I work together to create a tray depicting a problem and then take turns adding things to the tray, or taking things out of the tray, to show possible solutions to the problem (Kottman & Meany-Walen, 2016). I also use a sand tray in the fourth phase of therapy (reorientation/reeducation). For instance, sand tray work can help clients to express feelings and learn positive ways of viewing themselves, others, and the world. Sand trays can also metaphorically represent new contexts for the client to practice new behaviors and skills.

Robert Jason Grant, EdD, RPT-S

I implement traditional sand tray therapy work with my neurotypical clients. Much of this work is based on the work of Homeyer and Sweeney (2017) which defined sand tray therapy as "an expressive and projective mode of psychotherapy that has the unique and extraordinary quality of being considerably flexible and adaptive" (p. 6). It can integrate a variety of theoretical and technical psychotherapeutic approaches. It can be nondirective or directive, completely nonverbal or verbally assisted, and incorporate techniques from a wide spectrum of counseling approaches. I have a designated sand tray therapy room which has a standard sand tray and miniature display common to what would be found in most sand tray therapy setups. I have utilized this type of sand tray therapy for a variety of issues and with a variety of clients including children, teens, and adults.

I use sand trays for sensory work and as a skill development tool in working with children with autism. In sensory work, I offer the sand tray and other types of trays such as KayKob, beans, grass seed, and rice as sensory trays that the child can manipulate to help regulate their system and help with sensory input issues. I keep these trays on shelves in my playroom and children can access them as needed. If a child with autism is capable, I will use sand tray therapy without alterations, but I often use the sand tray as a skill development tool for children with autism, especially those who do not understand symbolic and pretend play. Often the focus is on improving social skills, regulation ability, and engagement and connection. In a skill development process, the sand tray becomes a tool to help increase the child's skill deficits. A child struggling with peer social interactions might participate in a turn-taking sand tray or creating a sand tray together to work on skills such as working with another person and being less rigid and controlling in play. A child struggling with connecting with another person might participate in some connection and engagement activities in the sand tray such as burying and unburying each other's hands in the sand or tracing each other's hands and fingers in the sand to help children with autism gain skills in becoming more comfortable being with and engaging with another person.

The sand tray is an active and present part of my playroom and therapy approach but can differ in its uses depending on the client. I might take a more traditional sand tray therapy approach or use a sand tray for sensory work or use the sand tray in implementing a structured intervention to work on skill development. The sand tray as an item in the playroom holds many possibilities for children. It may be accessed in a less formal or more formal way but certainly can be a valuable process in the playroom.

Heidi Gerard Kaduson, PhD, RPT-S

I am trained in Jungian and Gestalt sand play, but I do not have a sand tray in my main playroom. If I feel that a client needs sand tray work as the best approach for the individual client or if the client wants to do sand tray work,

I will take them into the sand tray room where there are miniatures and we can do a more formal sand tray therapy process. They are also welcome to use anything they have seen or need from the main playroom. I do not use sand tray therapy with every child client, but almost all young adults go to the sand tray room and show me their world.

Sand tray work has increased since I started using the Virtual Sandtray App (VSA). Because most children are so competent in iPad games, they really enjoy creating their worlds through this method. The variety of characters, scenes, atmospheres, places, and so on available in the VSA are innumerable. I couldn't possibly have the same amount and variety of miniatures in my sand tray room, and children gain so much freedom and confidence in building their sand trays through the VSA. Once they have finished, many children share their VSA creation with me, usually creating a narrative about their psychological difficulties.

Jennifer Lefebre, PsyD, RPT-S

One of my favorite ways to use a sand tray is during supervision or within my own self-care and processing of clients. I have offered the opportunity for supervisees to create a client's world, and then utilized a variety of process questions to look at the client and the supervisees experience of the client. New metaphors are often found, as well as different perspectives. The chance to process sessions or material that has posed as a challenge through a sand tray adds an element of distancing, which often leads to the ability to discover more about oneself as a play therapist. I often will create a sand tray at the end of the day to assist in my own self-care. I will take a picture of it and reflect on themes, and at times will bring it to my own supervision.

In the play therapy room with clients, the sand tray has been used as a sensory tool, with clients using a variety of different tools and toys to assist in regulation. Pouring, sifting, and feeling the sand, as well as making designs or tracing a labyrinth in the sand, are some of the ways many of the children I work with have used the sand tray to help themselves regulate or transition into session. Additionally, the burying and unburying of items, or their hands, is another way that children have used the sand tray to assist in developing object constancy, as well as to fulfil any sensory needs.

I often invite clients to create their calm/gentle/fantasy worlds in the sand tray. They will choose figures and nature items to create amazing worlds, and we then use our senses to make the worlds come alive (e.g., what would the temperature be – feel; what might we eat here – taste), in order to create a solid resource for them. I also use sand tray work quite frequently as an EMDR resource, in part for the creation of a safe place or container, but also may include more abstract mandalas or designs for centering and grounding, particularly with my adolescent or adult clients.

At times, I have been more directive and might ask clients to create a particular scene (i.e., their family doing something together, a school, the future), a piece of their experience, or a portion of their trauma narrative through a sand tray. I offer these with minimal prompting and watch and reflect as the process unfolds.

Clair Mellenthin, MSW, RPT-S

I am trained in sand tray therapy and utilize this therapeutic approach in my play therapy practice, rather than the Jungian model of sand play. Sand tray therapy has been defined as,

> … an expressive and projective mode of psychotherapy involving the unfolding and processing of intra- and inter-personal issues throughout the use of specific sandtray materials as a nonverbal medium of communication, led by the client or therapist and facilitated by a trained therapist.
> (Homeyer & Sweeney, 2017, p. 6)

The sand tray is typically both expressive and projective, as well as flexible and adaptive (Homeyer & Sweeney, 2017). I use the sand tray as an expressive therapy tool, as it allows for connection, processing, and self-discovery. As with all interventions, I tend to practice from an integrated theoretical approach. I have multiple sand trays available in my play therapy room that have different colors and textures of sand in them. I use sand tray therapy quite often in my play therapy work, with children, teens, and adults. I find it to be an invaluable tool in family and couple work as well. I tend to be predominantly nondirective in my use with the sand tray and allow this to be a tool for the child to use if they choose to. The sand tray and shelves of miniatures are in plain sight and located on a child-size table so that it is easily accessible to the youngest child.

I find that children utilize the sand tray in their play therapy process as a tool from everything to self-soothing and regulation to working through significant trauma and attachment issues. As with other expressive therapies, sand tray work gives words to the unspeakable as the child is able to create their world, their thoughts and feelings, and their experiences utilizing symbolism and metaphor. Through this work, a child can find their words and find their voice – even if no words are ever spoken.

I love using sand tray work in my play therapy supervision and often will have my graduate interns and supervisees create sand trays representing challenging case studies, review issues of transference and countertransference, as well as review their personal progression toward becoming a competent play therapist. I find this is an invaluable tool in the supervision process and it allows for personal reflection, insight, and awareness in both the supervisor and supervisee.

Akiko J. Ohnogi, PsyD

I believe that utilizing sand tray work in play therapy is extremely therapeutic. If a play therapist has the means to devote a room just for various sand trays,

I think that it would be important that they put thought into the designs of the trays, types of sand available, the miniatures, and how they are all positioned.

Apart from taking a semester course in graduate school and several sand tray workshops at professional conferences throughout the years, I have not had formal training in the use of sand tray therapy. Thus, my use of a sand tray is as one of the many toys and materials that can be used therapeutically in play, rather than a formalized version of conducting and interpreting the images created within the sand trays.

I have the sand tray in my play therapy room along with all the other toys and materials. I have many miniatures that can be included in the sand tray, as well as can be used in other activities as well. They are in plastic toy boxes sorted out by type (people, vehicles, animals, etc.), rather than displayed out in open cabinets.

The sand that I use is Kinetic Sand™ for sensory activities. Examples of this include running hands through the sand, creating different shapes in different sizes, and watching the sand slowly change shape. I also ask clients to create "My World" in the sand tray based on Lowenfeld's classic intervention (1997). I will follow the instruction for "My World" and invite the children to,

> Create your world, how you define it and how to design it, is up to you. Use the sand and tray however you would like. You can use any of the miniatures, toys, and other material to create your world. Then, you can take away or rearrange objects to make your world better. Next, you can take away or rearrange that which interferes with making it better. Now, you can take away or rearrange objects to counteract or protect your world from the interferences. Lastly, finish your world the way you would like it to be right now, before we end the session.

I discuss each creation after the client has completed the instruction, before moving on with the next prompt.

Mary Anne Peabody, EdD, RPT-S

I use sand tray therapy both as a directive and nondirective modality and find it to be one of the most versatile modalities across age ranges. My work in sand tray therapy is informed by Homeyer and Sweeney's (2017) six-step protocol depending on my therapeutic intention with individual children or their family. I would describe my selection of miniatures as minimal, as I find too many miniatures overwhelming for both children and for me. Decades ago, I invested in the original natural, burnt orange–hued *Jurassic Sand*, *www.jurassicsand.com* and I have never used another type of sand. My sand tray is large enough for me to sit on the floor next to a child or across from them.

When my treatment plan calls for a nondirective play therapy approach, my sand tray and miniatures are offered as one of the many choices in the playroom space. If the treatment calls for an integrative approach I may begin treatment utilizing a child-centered play therapy orientation (Landreth, 2012) and over time move into Adlerian play therapy (Kottman & Meany-Walen, 2016) structuring the sand tray therapy process more with directive prompts to assess early recollections, lifestyle conceptualization, identify family atmosphere, or in the reeducation or reorientation phase of treatment.

Additionally, I regularly use sand tray therapy in play therapy supervision to enhance self-awareness and professional growth (Bratton et al., 2008; Morrison & Homeyer, 2008). I was fortunate to be trained by Marijane Fall and Jack Sutton (2004) who used sand tray therapy modalities in our "supervision of supervision" coursework and practicum experiences and have been greatly influenced by the power of sand tray work during clinical supervision.

Dee Ray, PhD, RPT-S

In child-centered play therapy, I have a sandbox in the playroom which children use in myriad ways, including as a sand tray for fluid play scenes. When children build a scene in the sandbox, I attempt to understand their world through empathic reflections of feeling, content, and themes. I do not use prompts to structure their scenes or processing questions to provide insight because this type of structuring seems developmentally inappropriate for younger children.

I do use the more typical form of sand tray work in therapy with older children/preadolescents, adults, and often in supervision with play therapists. From my perspective, sand tray work is one of the least threatening expressive arts to use with adults who sometimes tend to be hesitant with creative expressions of experiences. The containment of the sand in a tray and the use of formed figures appears to reduce the older client's resistance to engaging in a symbolic experience. As with most expressive arts, I start with a broad (e.g., create a scene in the sand) or narrow prompt (e.g., make scene of you with your friends at school) depending upon the client's situation. I also enjoy using sand tray in groupwork. I may ask clients in a group to make individual trays that we process and attempt to bridge commonalities or to make a group tray in which we explore group dynamics. In supervision, I use sand tray to help play therapists explore their self-concept in the context of their client relationships (e.g., make a scene of you as a therapist), their relationship with certain clients (e.g., make a scene of you with the client we were just talking about), or their work-life balance (e.g., make a scene of you at both work and home). In all sand tray activities, I seek to explore the experience through processing observations of the person's approach to making the scene, the person's perception of their scene, and the person's emotional reactions to the experience.

Jessica Stone, PhD, RPT-S

Gisela DeDomenico, PhD, elevated my understanding and respect for sand tray therapy during a training in 2003. Prior to learning and experiencing sand tray through Dr. Domenico's approach, sand tray was something I knew about but didn't fully understand. Since that time, I have been to numerous trainings with people I respect greatly and have read works by Margaret Lowenfeld to "hear" from the master herself. The sand tray is an amazingly powerful tool, and one must continue to seek knowledge and experience through it.

My office has a traditional sand tray setup with open shelving for my miniatures/symbols. The shelves are organized with like items grouped together. There is a sense of satisfaction watching clients peruse the shelving looking for the item that "speaks" to them and the creation they are making. The worlds created are to be deeply respected and honored as revealing invitations into one's inner experience.

The sand tray is utilized in my office with a primarily nondirective approach. Clients know the sand tray setup is in the playroom as it is prominent. In addition, each client is given a tour and description of the items in the room when they initially present for services. At times, it is deemed appropriate to employ a more directive approach with clients depending on their needs. In this case, a client might be asked to create a tray with a particular experience or theme in mind.

I have both a traditional sand tray and virtual sand tray available in my office for use by people of all ages. The Virtual Sandtray App (Stone, 2015) was born out of a recognized need and further developed as the identified uses multiplied. During the 2011 tsunami disaster in Japan, a dear friend and colleague, Dr. Akiko Ohnogi, put out a plea on Facebook for help with materials so that she and her colleagues could help those affected. After I collected items and sent them to Japan, I remarked to my husband that I could not see how they would use the sand tray with the people they were readying to help. This felt like a lost opportunity to me, as in, the sand tray could be a very powerful tool in this situation and it would not be available. I started to think about the ways it could be truly portable and suddenly it hit me, a tablet. After some time the Virtual Sandtray App was born.

The Virtual Sandtray App for tablets and VR allows another experience in sand tray therapy for anyone to use but are particularly helpful with people who are unable or unwilling to participate in the traditional form for a variety of reasons. For some, the tactile experience of the sand is precisely why they will not use sand tray. For others, the sensory experience might be overwhelming, such as those with significant trauma histories. Some people who have motor difficulties or need assistance in moving could find a traditional tray to be very difficult or impossible to use. Others might be in environments where a traditional tray setup is not possible or convenient, such as hospitals, home visits, facilities, and disaster sites. The Virtual Sandtray App increases the accessibility to this amazing tool for many different people. In addition, it capitalizes on the client's generational interest and desire to use digital tools. Highly motivating activities will yield higher compliance and increased engagement.

Daniel Sweeney, PhD, RPT-S

Sand tray therapy is a big part of my play therapy work. My approach is detailed in Homeyer and Sweeney (2017) and Sweeney (2016). However, in response to the wording of this question, I need to make an important distinction. Unlike the majority of my colleagues, I do <u>not</u> include the classic [20″ × 30″] sand tray in my play therapy room; rather, I have a large [36″ × 36″] sandbox in my playroom.

I rarely use sand tray therapy with young children. I use a sand tray with preadolescents, adolescents, and adults. I have found my primarily CCPT approach with young children and filial therapy (Landreth & Bratton, 2020) with parents to be quite effective. Also, I tend to be more cognitive and directive in my sand tray therapy work, which is inconsistent with my approach to working with young children.

Additionally, my collection of sand tray miniatures is extensive, and I prefer to keep this separate from my more "traditional" play therapy room. I rarely have to set limits on being destructive or making a mess of my miniature collection with older youth – whereas in the playroom, children are free to completely empty the shelves of toys.

Thus, my use of sand tray therapy with children is the exception, not the norm. Some children will use the sandbox in a sand tray therapy–like manner, but I do not direct them to do so. Also, whereas I use the classic "tracking" responses in the playroom, I generally do not track in the sand tray therapy process.

References

Bainum, C. R., Schneider, M. F., & Stone, M. H. (2006). An Adlerian model for sandtray therapy. *The Journal of Individual Psychology, 62*, 36–46.

Bratton, S., Ceballos, P., & Sheely, A. (2008). Use of expressive arts in a humanistic approach to play therapy supervision: Facilitating supervisee self-awareness. In A. A. Drewes & J. Mullen (Eds.), *Supervision can be playful: Techniques for child and play therapist supervisors* (pp. 211–232). Jason Aronson.

Carey, L. (1990). Sandplay therapy with a troubled child. *The Arts in Psychotherapy, 17*, 197–209.

Fall, M., & Sutton, J. M. Jr. (2004). *Clinical supervision: A handbook for practitioners.* Allyn & Bacon.

Homeyer, L. E., & Sweeney, D. S. (2017). *Sandtray therapy: A practical manual* (3rd ed.) Routledge.

Kottman, T., & Meany-Walen, K. (2016). *Partners in play: An Adlerian approach to play therapy* (3rd ed.). American Counseling Association.

Landreth, G. L. (2012). *Play therapy: The art of the relationship* (3rd ed.). Brunner-Routledge.

Landreth, G. L., & Bratton, S. (2020). *Child-parent relationship therapy (CPRT): An evidence-based 10-session filial therapy model* (2nd ed.). Routledge.

Lowenfeld, M. (1997). *Understanding children's sandplay: Lowenfeld's world technique.* Sussex Academic Press.

Morrison, M., & Homeyer, L. E. (2008). Supervision in the sand. In A. A. Drewes & J. A. Mullen (Eds.). *Supervision can be playful: Techniques for child and play therapist supervisors* (pp. 233–248). Jason Aronson.

Stone, J. (2015). *Virtual Sandtray App.* https://www.sandtrayplay.com/Press/Virtual-SandtrayArticle01.pdf.

Sweeney, D. (2016). Sandtray therapy: A neurobiological approach. In E. Prendiville & J. Howard (Eds.), *Creative psychotherapy: Applying the principles of neurobiology to play and expressive arts-based practice.* Routledge.

13 How Do You Use Expressive Arts in Play Therapy?

Jeff Ashby, PhD, RPT-S

I use expressive arts in play therapy in much the same way I use sand tray work. My guiding theoretical perspective (AdPT) allows for a broad eclecticism of technique in the service of therapeutic ends (Kottman & Meany-Walen, 2016). Similar to sand tray work, expressive arts can be used as a projective; a window into the child's inner world. My experience is that some children are drawn to the expressive arts. They are naturally drawn to the art supplies in the playroom and, when engaged in nondirected play, gravitate to them ("pipe cleaners, glitter, and glue – Oh My!"). In the same way that a sand tray is a possible medium for assessment and intervention, I view expressive arts in the same way. I generally assess a client's interest and enthusiasm for expressive arts early in therapy, often using a kinetic family drawing to begin to assess family constellation and atmosphere (Knoff & Prout, 1985). However, if I am already aware that a client may not enjoy drawing, I may ask the child to create a kinetic family sand tray, or collage (cutting and pasting pictures and words from magazines and other sources to depict the family).

One of the things I love about play therapy is the ability to tailor assessment and interventions to individual clients. As a result, no play therapy process looks the same. This is plainly illustrated for me in the use of expressive arts in therapy. There are clients who engage with expressive arts in all four phases of therapy. They are doing kinetic family drawings, making sculptures depicting their strengths and assets, illustrating and laminating pages to make into books about their experience, and on and on. There are other clients for whom expressive arts hold no attraction. For those clients, the course of therapy looks very different.

One of the values of expressive arts is the nonverbal expression of the child's inner world. I want to understand the child's lifestyle, their feelings, beliefs, attitudes, and concerns. Expressive arts are one way for clients to communicate these preconscious, subconscious, and unconscious aspects of themselves. Expressive arts also offer me a way to meet the client where they are and help facilitate insight and reorientation. In the third or fourth phase of therapy, I might use O'Connor's (1983) Color-Your-Life technique to help clients identify and understand various affective states. However, for a child who is less interested in expressive arts, I might use McDowell's (1997) Pick-Up-Sticks Game, structured to accomplish the same therapeutic goal. Like sand tray work, kinetic movement, and music – expressive arts are one of several possible mediums through which to intervene and assess (it's just often messier – as glitter can get everywhere …).

Robert Jason Grant, EdD, RPT-S

Expressive arts, creative play, play, art, and play interventions – the distinctive differences between these constructs can become blurry. It is challenging to universally define what is meant by expressive arts in play therapy. For purposes of a general definition, expressive arts in therapy with children can be thought of as a process that combines psychology and creative processes to promote emotional growth and healing. It is an integrative approach in psychological or counseling therapy that can include using music, dance, drama, poetry, drawing, finger painting, movement, clay, and Play-Doh creation, and many different creative materials to explore and express.

I appreciate and value the ability for children to enter the playroom and be able to create and express in any way that feels comfortable for them. To this end, I make sure to have several expressive materials and toys available in the playroom for children to access. This would include but not limited to dress up clothes, masks, hats, clay, Play-Doh, paint, drawing materials, music instruments, space for movement, and various creation materials such as pipe cleaners, various paper, craft sticks, and beads. These toys and materials are always present for children to access in a nondirective manner and I also use expressive materials in directive play therapy interventions that I might implement with a child. Some children enjoy engaging in expressive arts more than others. I try to be mindful of the child and what he or she prefers and enjoys when selecting directive interventions involving expressive arts.

I once worked with a preadolescent girl who had been diagnosed with Asperger's syndrome and sensory processing disorder. In learning about her and her preferences, I discovered that she hated movement-based activities and processes, she also disliked drama and role play activities. She loved creating in more traditional ways such as drawing and painting. I introduced the *Sensory Mandala* intervention (Grant, 2018) to her. This intervention involves creating a mandala using various tactile and olfactory sensory materials. It became a favorite and one she used at home to help her improve regulation ability. She loved creating sensory mandalas and when she felt she need some regulating work at home, she would go into her room and create a sensory mandala. The process spoke to her and gave her a regulation tool. In some ways this reminds me of another question in this book – How do you speak the client's language? Allowing this child to be herself and access what was meaningful and fulfilling to her created change. Letting her language be spoken and not trying to change it facilitated growth for her. Even the introduction of a specific directive intervention was based on understanding and respecting her preferences and what was meaningful to her.

Heidi Gerard Kaduson, PhD, RPT-S

I use expressive arts most of the time – especially in trauma related cases – and usually when the child begins latency age around 9–12 years and older. I have everything they need, so I will follow their lead regarding the medium. I will ask the client to draw a picture of a person, house, tree, and family during intake, and after that, they can do what they prefer. If the request for these drawings is met with disdain from children, I will avoid it. If they show a lot of anxiety while drawing (erasing a lot, tiny bricks all over the house, etc.), I will tell them that it's "good enough", and "let's play". I work with all children and adults through metaphors, so I follow what they are doing or making and find a metaphor or metaphors that can be directly used in the play therapy treatment.

I have created many new expressive art techniques just to fit certain types of children who seem lost – incapable of pretend play and stuck without being able to use typical expressive art materials. The *Sticker Story* has been one of the most successful interventions for very bright children whose social and emotional levels are much lower than their cognitive ability. In introducing this intervention, I give the child a piece of paper that I have folded into 6 boxes. I label the three columns as "friends", "school" and "family". The top row of each section is for positive representations and the bottom of each section is for the negative representations. They are then provided with boxes of stickers that they can peruse and choose stickers that seem to fit each of the boxes on the paper. It can take an entire session for gifted teens to do this because my clients enjoy searching and gathering what they need. When the client's sticker story is finished, they look it over and tell me what it says to them. It isn't the telling of the story that is most therapeutic for the children but the actual process of sorting through and deciding what to pick for each of the boxes. Gifted teenagers gain so much insight into their own psychological self by doing this technique, and most of them finish the sticker story and are able to then communicate verbally about their difficulties. Expressive arts can also produce the beginning of trauma work when we ask a child to "show me" what happened. Since trauma is housed in the right hemisphere of the brain, bringing colorful materials and mediums to use allows a child to slowly go back and remember parts of the traumatic event – assimilating small amounts of that knowledge at their own pace. In some cases, where a child is not able to begin through expressive arts, I use cognitive behavioral play therapy techniques like *Color Your Heart* (Kaduson, 2006) to get them into the play or to hopefully aide in the expression of feelings and underlying difficulties.

Jennifer Lefebre, PsyD, RPT-S

I view the expressive arts therapies as an essential part of play therapy. I believe all forms of creativity are essential to the healing process, and when combined with the understanding of the therapeutic powers of play, magic can happen!

Art, music, movement/yoga, dance, and drama all have formalized creative strategies founded in theories of psychotherapy, to create rich resources for individuals of all ages (Malchiodi, 2005). In this regard, I am often able to introduce or connect with clients who might have been hesitant to engage in play therapy by using the expressive therapies.

There are several family and individual drawing techniques that I use during my initial intake and when assessing a client or family. Many children enjoy making masks, collages, models, and dioramas in the play therapy room as well. I've had many children request to make slime or oobleck as a way to self-regulate, and expressive therapy techniques have been particularly helpful with children who have been sexually abused, those who are encopretic or enuretic, and those who engage in self-injurious behaviors such as cutting. When doing parts work or exploring deeper shadow work, I have used black paper to trace shadows or made shadow boxes to further explore these areas. Shadow work is very challenging and can be a very emotional process. Expressive therapy techniques are a wonderful way to support this process. Shadow work is a form of examining oneself through the parts we keep hidden from the world, facing that which takes great strength and will, in turn, lead to significant emotional growth.

Music is one of my favorite things for my own self-care, and I often use it in the therapeutic process. Creating play lists with clients for different emotions or experiences, using singing games with a family, or playing freeze dance are ways that I integrate music into play therapy. Movement and dance seem to naturally flow when music is involved, and I utilize trauma-sensitive yoga as part of this as well. These activities assist in regulation and attunement and can also facilitate attachment amongst family members.

I have a young adult I am working with who played a song for me and we watched the video. We had a rich discussion of how the lyrics pertained to their life and how they could use the music to help battle suicidal ideation and self-injurious thoughts. We created a dance move that went along with the song and drew out the main lyric that stood out, even thinking about it as a potential tattoo. This also led to the creation of a container to "hold their demons" and a visual representation of the container was made. This young adult created a calm place through the sand tray, adding the container and various symbols and figures that were representations of the song. This is one of my favorite case examples of how I integrate the expressive arts into my work.

Clair Mellenthin, MSW, RPT-S

I use expressive arts frequently in play therapy. In my playroom, we have an expressive arts station that consists of bins of craft items such as popsicle sticks, glitter, googly eyes, pipe cleaners, magazines for collage, pom-poms, stickers, paint, glue, string, and beads. These are neatly organized and easily accessible for children young and old. By approaching play therapy with a prescriptive approach, it allows for the tailoring of the therapy sessions to the individual needs of the client. I utilize both directive and nondirective approaches when using expressive arts, as it depends on the treatment needs of the client.

Expressive arts can be a powerful tool in your play therapy toolbox. Expressive arts help clients of all ages "gain a better understanding of themselves, achieve higher awareness of behavior patterns, and gain greater concentration and learning capabilities as well as fulfill the human needs for self-expression" (Perryman, Moss, & Cochran, 2015, p. 207). When utilizing the creative process, this can help to decrease defense mechanisms, access the unconscious, and give words to the unspeakable. Eaton, Doherty, and Widrick (2007) stated, "Creative expression provides a means by which the child can express experiences, memories, and emotions that he or she may not be able to put into words" (p. 261).

I find that the process of creating can be a powerful experience and allows time for quiet and reflection, as well as act as a vehicle to process the experience and the symbolic representations the client has discovered. Externalizing confusing inner experiences within an active play or creative therapeutic process can facilitate a child's sequencing their "storyline" or life story, while "engaging more fully with sensory and somatic experiences, becoming more aware of their own bodily sensations, and developing insight into how they process emotions" (Prendiville, 2014, p. 87).

Akiko J. Ohnogi, PsyD

I have a variety of expressive arts materials along with toys for clients to use if/when they would like and in any way they would like. If I assess that a structured activity will be useful and necessary, I often instruct the client in an activity using expressive arts materials. I find that expressive arts utilized in play therapy are an extremely powerful therapeutic means of psychological treatment, especially for clients working on healing from trauma.

The following are some examples of the structured activities I use with expressive arts. These interventions focus on emotional aspects of the healing process. Focusing on emotions and talking about the creations helps with cognitive understanding of the issues and leads to behavioral change in the child.

- *My Dragon*: Instruct the child to create a dragon out of clay or Play-Doh which symbolizes their specific fear/anxiety. Ask the child to give it a name and describe its characteristics. The child is asked to make things that will make the dragon more powerful, and something that can fight against it. The child is invited to create things to strengthen this tool and can fight the dragon, as well as things that will interfere with the fighting. This process is done over several sessions, with the child changing, adding, and taking away from their symbols and objects as their fear/anxiety decreases.
- *My Life*: This is a collage created to instill hope. The child is provided with various art and craft materials and magazines to cut and paste onto

a large piece of construction paper (the color of paper is the client's choice). The child will create a collage titled "My Life". They are instructed to include in the collage things they consider a problem, as well as things that can help, protect, provide a sense of security, and enhance positive feelings. The child is given permission to add, change, or take away from the collage to combat the problem and increase the supportive factors.

- *Good Luck Charm*: This is a drawing made to symbolize safety/protection. Ask the child to choose two sheets of construction paper, one in their favorite color and the other paper their least favorite color. The child chooses something to draw with (crayon, markers, colored pencil), one is a color they like the other a color they do not like. Instruct the child to draw on their least favorite colored paper something that is a problem for them, using the "dislike" color drawing implement. The child is invited to draw on the favorite colored paper things that make them happy, excited, calm, and/or feel safe and protected, with the "like" color. The child rips up the problem paper while chanting out loud or silently a mantra that the child creates (e.g., "*problem* go away", "I hate you *problem*"). The child stomps on the torn pieces of paper and throws them away. The child then folds the protective paper into a small piece and writes/draws name on one side and "good luck charm" on the other side. The child keeps the good luck charm and takes it home.

Mary Anne Peabody, EdD, RPT-S

I consider expressive arts in play therapy when I combine toys with art materials (drawing, painting, puppets, clay, visual pictures, LEGO bricks, sand tray) to extend the theory being utilized. I believe that most play therapy theories can be successfully enhanced by expressive arts interventions. All forms of play, art, music making, dance, drama, and creative writing require participatory energy and are sensory-rich experiences (Malchiodi, 2015). Whether it is visual, auditory, or kinetic, children and adults appear to benefit and explore into areas where words alone may be inadequate.

Expressive arts often seem to deepen and expedite the therapeutic process. This notion is echoed by Gladding (2012) as he suggests using the expressive arts may speed up the process of externalization allowing people to experience themselves differently. My own research with LEGO bricks supports this finding (Peabody & Noyes, 2017).

I use a variety of expressive arts for assessment purposes informed by Gil's approach to extended play-based developmental assessment (Gil, 2015). By utilizing expressive arts early in the process, children and parents are quickly exposed to how I value and will use play as the key driver in my treatment delivery. I also use expressive materials during family play therapy (Czyszczon et al., 2015; Gil, 2015) as I believe many parents need more playtime in their lives and expressive arts can provide a sensory-rich opportunity.

Naturally the supervision of play therapists lends itself to experiential techniques as play therapy is characteristically experiential. I believe it is the supervisor's responsibility to consider the supervisee's developmental level, supervisee characteristics, and ethical concerns when choosing expressive arts activities (Purswell & Stulmaker, 2015). Our tools are powerful and must be intentionally selected. This holistic sensitivity to the powerful process of expressive arts in supervision honors the supervisory relationship and the process itself.

Dee Ray, PhD, RPT-S

As a child-centered play therapist, I provide traditional child-centered play therapy to children between the ages of 3 and 10 years old, meaning that I provide materials in the playroom in which the child can play in a self-directed manner without structure imposed by the play therapist. In the natural course of development, children acquire advanced cognitive and verbal skills that allow them to express themselves beyond the language of play. Expressive arts provide a therapeutic modality for older children to integrate their new verbal and cognitive abilities with their fluent language of play. For adolescents and adults, expressive arts allow the person who has become disconnected from play to access symbolic expression and reconnect with processes out-of-awareness. When I work with children who are approximately 9–10 years old, I will consider introducing expressive arts structured activities to assess the child's preference for self-directed play versus an external prompt for a play activity. If the child seems constrained or acquiescent to my prompt, I typically move to the facilitation of self-directed play because they appear to still operate in the primary language of play. As they mature, preadolescents often prefer prompts in order to blend their need for verbal and play expression.

Expressive arts activities are essential to my work with preadolescents, adolescents, and adults. They provide the connection to play so desperately needed as people grow older and experience limited access to their emotions. However, I am careful to use expressive arts intentionally and based in a consistent theoretical orientation. Degges-White and Davis (2018) provide a helpful understanding of approaching expressive arts from an intentional framework to counseling. I am also deliberate in selecting expressive arts mediums that pair well with clients and provide a safe outlet for the individual client. I find Landgarten's (1987) continuum of least controlled (most threatening for clients) to most controlled (least threatening) materials for expressive arts to be helpful in my decision-making regarding the introduction of activities. For clients who see themselves as lacking creativity or artistic ability, I will start with simple materials like paper, pencils, and markers while other clients respond well to clay and more organic materials. I use both broad prompts (e.g., create your world) and narrow prompts (e.g., make a scene of your family at Thanksgiving) depending on the client's characteristics and goals.

When teaching expressive arts, I emphasize the art and skill of processing the activity over the doing of the activity. The relational, insight, and change elements of expressive arts activities typically take place in the processing of the activity, both internal and external processing. Play therapists sometimes become caught up in the excitement of the activity itself and neglect to facilitate reflection and support of the client. At the end of an activity, I engage in processing questions, reflections of content, feelings, and patterns, and facilitation of client's exploration of their experience. For me, relational processing is the essential reason for engaging in expressive arts.

Jessica Stone, PhD, RPT-S

Expressive arts are very popular amongst play therapists. I have many materials in my office for use, such as different art media, paper types, sensory water beads, artificial snow, and items to create personal books, calming jars, and slime. I have, at times, brought in ingredients to mix and bake with clients.

Included in these expressive arts materials is a virtual reality headset. Programs such as Tilt Brush and SculptVR allow the client to create amazing artistic scenes and worlds in immersive, interactive, three-dimensional form. A variety of apps for tablets, such as Bubbles, Fluidity, and Morfo, allow for another way to express creatively.

Coming from a prescriptive viewpoint, the needs of the client will dictate the items used within the play therapy sessions. At times the sensory experience of some items will soothe and comfort, at times they will elicit important responses, and at times they will overwhelm. Expressive art materials must be used with conscientiousness and respect for the needs of the client within the play therapy process.

Many play therapy trainings include experiential exercises where the play therapist is creating some type of craft. People in these trainings are often having a lot of fun creating the item(s). I think an important focus for our field is to ensure that the practice of the creation is to increase the familiarity both with the mechanics of the creation and with whatever potential responses the activity could activate in a client. At times it seems the exercises within trainings become more about the therapist than the client and we should be cautious. If the focus is for self-awareness or other things the therapist needs to process, then it should be labeled as such without issue.

Daniel Sweeney, PhD, RPT-S

It is important to define what is meant by the term "expressive arts". Malchiodi (2015) contends that "Expressive therapies are defined as the use of art, music, drama, dance/movement, poetry/creative writing, bibliotherapy, play, and/or sandplay within the context of psychotherapy, counseling, rehabilitation, or medicine" (p. 12). Malchiodi goes on to state that "creative arts therapies and expressive therapies are not merely subsets of play therapy and have a long history as distinct approaches in mental health and health care" (p. 13). I agree with her and would say that play therapy belongs under the umbrella of "expressive therapies", and not the other way around.

I am not a registered art therapist [ATR (Art Therapy Credentials Board)] or registered expressive arts therapist [REAT (International Expressive Arts Therapy Association)], and never attempt to purport that I am, just as I would never want someone to promote being an RPT when they are not. I do use, however, art therapy techniques and various expressive arts interventions.

The primary expressive arts approach that I use as a play therapist is sand tray therapy. Homeyer and Sweeney (2017) define sand tray therapy as

> an expressive and projective mode of psychotherapy involving the unfolding and processing of intra- and inter-personal issues through the use of specific sandtray materials as a nonverbal medium of communication, led by the client or therapist and facilitated by a trained therapist.
>
> (p. 6)

The expressive and projective qualities of sand tray therapy apply to most expressive arts interventions.

I use a variety of expressive arts interventions, in addition to play therapy and sand tray therapy. These include such interventions as Play-Doh/clay work, painting and drawing, art-based genograms, therapeutic storytelling, puppet plays, dollhouse play, mandalas, drama, poetry, creative writing/journaling, bibliotherapy, and others.

References

Czyszczon, G., Riviere, S., Lowman, D. K., & Stewart, A. L. (2015). Family play therapy: Practical techniques. In D. A. Crenshaw & A. L. Stewart (Eds.), *Play therapy: A comprehensive guide to theory and practice*. Guilford Press.

Degges-White, S., & Davis, N. (Eds.). (2018). *Integrating expressive arts into counseling practice: Theory-based interventions* (2nd ed.). Springer.

Eaton, G., Doherty, K., & Widrick, R. (2007). A review of research and methods used to establish art therapy as an effective treatment method for traumatized children. *Child & Adolescent Psychiatry, 15*(1), 52–55.

Gill, E. (2015). *Play in family therapy*. Guilford Press.

Gladding, S. T. (2012). Art in counseling. In C. A. Malchiodi (Ed.), *Handbook of art therapy* (2nd ed., pp. 263–274). Guilford Press.

Grant, R. J. (2018). *Understanding sensory processing challenges: A workbook for children and teens*. AutPlay Publishing.

Homeyer, L., & Sweeney, D. (2017). *Sandtray therapy: A practical manual* (3rd ed.). Routledge.

Kaduson, H. G. (2006). Release play therapy for children with post-traumatic stress order. In H. G. Kaduson & C. E. Schaefer (Eds.), *Short-term play therapy for children* (2nd ed., pp. 3–22). Guilford.

Kottman, T., & Meany-Walen, K. (2016). *Partners in play: An Adlerian approach to play therapy* (3rd ed.). American Counseling Association.

Kaduson, H., & Schaefer, C. (Eds.). (1997). *101 favorite play therapy techniques*. Jason Aronson.

Knoff, H., & Prout, H. (1985). *Kinetic drawing system for family and school: A handbook*. Western Psychological Services.

Landgarten, H. (1987). *Family art psychotherapy: A clinical guide and casebook*. Brunner/Mazel.

Malchiodi, C. A. (2005). *Expressive therapies*. Guilford Press.

Malchiodi, C. A. (2015). Neurobiology, creative interventions and childhood trauma. In C. A. Malchiodi (Ed.), *Creative interventions with traumatized children* (2nd ed., pp. 3–23). Guilford Publications.

McDowell, B. (1997). The pick-up sticks game. In H. Kaduson & C. E. Schaefer (Eds.), *101 favorite play therapy techniques* (pp. 145–149). Jason Aronson.

O'Connor, K. J. (1983). The color-your-life technique. In C. E. Schaefer & K. J. O'Connor (Eds.), *Handbook of play therapy* (pp. 251–258). Wiley.

Peabody, M. A. & Noyes, S. (2017). Reflective boot camp: Adapting LEGO SERIOUS PLAY in higher education. *Reflective Practice: International and Multidisciplinary Perspectives*, 18(2), 232–243.

Perryman, K. L., Moss, R., & Cochran, K. (2015). Child-centered expressive arts and play therapy: School groups for at-risk adolescent girls. *International Journal of Play Therapy*, 24(4), 205–220.

Prendiville, E. (2014). Abreaction. In C. E. Schaefer & A. A. Drewes (Eds.), *The therapeutic powers of play* (pp. 83–102). Wiley.

Purswell, K. E., & Stulmaker, H. L. (2015). Expressive arts in supervision: Choosing developmentally appropriate interventions. *International Journal of Play Therapy*, 24(2), 103–107.

14 How Do You Address Issues of Intersectionality in Your Practice?

Jeff Ashby, PhD, RPT-S

The theory of intersectionality has a complex intellectual history that both complements and contrasts with traditional multiculturalism, standpoint theory, and multicultural feminist thought (e.g., Hancock, 2016). Among the complexities include whether intersectionality is a way to conceptualize multiple identities or is, instead, a framework for critiquing systemic and interacting forms of oppression and privilege (Grzanka et al., 2017). The intellectual terrain is further complicated for me by the need for "responsible stewardship of intersectionality" and "guidelines" for its responsible use (Moradi & Grzanka, 2017, p. 64).

Understanding intersectionality as the acknowledgement of holding multiple interacting identities is consistent with the Adlerian maxim that people are socially embedded (Carlson et al., 2005) and best understood in the context of their social networks and culture. While a number of authors have highlighted the effectiveness of AdPT with diverse groups (e.g., Herring & Runion, 1994), the intersection of multiple identities and their related framework of interacting forms of oppression has not been fully addressed. This represents a significant challenge for me as I work with refugee children and other traditionally marginalized groups and consistently work to understand the multidimensionality of their experience, rather than view them from a single-axis perspective (Crenshaw, 1989).

Ultimately, I would argue that actively addressing issues of intersectionality is consistent with Adler's (Ansbacher & Ansbacher, 1956) assertion that clinicians should treat the whole person. This is manifested in the playroom and in parental and teacher consultation. I take care to consider how intersecting cultural factors may influence the ways children express themselves through play, the sorts of systemic oppression and discrimination they (and their families) may be experiencing, the formulation of their goals and ideas about the world, and the responses they may have to different play therapy interventions.

Robert Jason Grant, EdD, RPT-S

The term "intersectionality" seems to have been coined by Kimberlé Crenshaw, law professor and social theorist, in her 1989 paper "Demarginalizing The Intersection of Race and Sex: A Black Feminist Critique of Antidiscrimination

Doctrine, Feminist Theory and Antiracist Politics". Intersectional theory asserts that people are often disadvantaged by multiple sources of oppression: their race, class, gender identity, sexual orientation, religion, and other identity markers. These markers do not exist independently of each other. Someone could potentially be affected (often in the form of oppression) by having multiple markers.

In play therapy, the purpose of looking at intersectionality as a theory would be to identify how clients in one or overlapping categories of identity are impacted and take these relationships into account when providing play therapy. I believe this could be addressed in multiple ways. Awareness and sensitivity on the part of the play therapists would be a good place to start. Implementing policy and protocol that supports respecting individuals would follow. My clinic recently updated our intake forms to reflect language that respects a person's gender preference, culture, and religious views. It is an easy task to update forms, and this simple change communicates to new clients they are entering an atmosphere of understanding and acceptance.

I often find myself in positions of advocating for individuals with disabilities and speaking about overt and sometimes nonpurposeful acts of oppression to those who have a disability. In my work as a trainer, I have had the opportunity to travel around the United States. I have been surprised by the number of therapy offices and clinics I have seen that are not handicap accessible. Often, I find bathrooms that are not handicap accessible, playrooms and offices that are upstairs in a building with no elevators, no handicap parking, no ramps to access the building entrance, and other setups that would not be accessible for many with disabilities. Many of these situations are a violation of the Americans with Disabilities Act (ADA) in the United States, yet they are still happening. I assume most of these oversights are innocent but the message to those with a disability is a rejecting one – because of your disability you are not welcome and/or cannot access mental health services here.

I try to maintain a place of staying open and continuing to offer better services and a therapeutic experience that will welcome individuals, empathize with their positions and situations, provide acceptance, accessibility, and unconditional positive regard, This is an ongoing process, but at least maintaining a mindset of trying to be aware will go a long way in addressing intersectionality issues.

Heidi Gerard Kaduson, PhD, RPT-S

I try to get all the information from the parents or caregivers regarding their cultural, religious, gender, etc., in the intake with the caregivers. I will ask specifically about traditions, general feelings of current issues that are socially prevalent, and so on. I do believe that there is bias and discrimination throughout our lives and certainly that can also be expressed or interpreted when people are in therapy. It is respectful and ethical to learn all that one can about the culture of the client and the family of the client. I make no judgment calls, and if I am not equipped with the clear understanding of the issues of intersectionality, then I might refer them to someone who might be a better match. I do not see everyone being treated equally or even fairly, but I totally believe that our treatment of children needs to be prescriptive – tailoring our treatment to their needs. Therefore, we need to ask, research, question, and maintain an open mind about anything that might be played out in the play therapy session.

The one common goal I usually have is to make sure that the client is thinking rationally (except if the client is in the preoperational stage of development where irrational thinking is normal) and then work with cognitive behavioral techniques to help the client to counter his or her irrational thoughts. Play therapists, as well as people in general, must study the varying levels of power and privilege that come with varying identities. Because we are play therapists, we are more likely to see children's perception of what their caregivers think or feel about these various issues. It is important, therefore, to work with the children and caregivers to respect their understanding of power and privilege and have their input as to what is important for the children and family. Once again, keeping an open mind, without judgment, and allowing new information to help us will only benefit the therapist's ability to help others.

Jennifer Lefebre, PsyD, RPT-S

Most clinical training programs include formal instruction in human diversity and cultural competence. Until recent years, the message of such training typically focused on developing an understanding about the client who is "diverse", and how they may progress in psychotherapy, and not about the therapist themselves. When cultural competence is viewed in terms of self-identity and self-awareness, there can be a shift in understanding the realities of human differences. Play therapy is the natural language of children, transcending language and ethnic barriers, thus offering creative responses to build strengths and resiliencies across cultures, allowing for the therapeutic powers of play to facilitate, initiate, and strengthen change (Drewes, 2005). Although it can be a challenge to maintain a culturally conscious and racially responsive stance when considering an individual's experiences and social identity within the context of discrimination and systemic inequities, play therapy allows for an avenue to heal and support these experiences.

My practice is a holistic trauma center in northwestern Connecticut which integrates psychotherapy, yoga, play therapy, and expressive arts therapies into the treatment of complex trauma. I built my practice in the community that I grew up in, which is a predominately Caucasian semirural area. I chose to build my practice here for several reasons, the main one is that this community is a big part of my self-identity. I was given the book *Limbo* (Lubrano, 2005) by one of my supervisors when I was on my way to my doctoral internship. My father is a machinist and my mother is a medical secretary, and I went to a trade school for high school so that I could work as a certified nurse's aide while putting myself through college. During my first practicum, I was reprimanded by my supervisor for not dressing professionally. I was wearing khaki pants and a nice sweater, but it was expected that I wear a suit, and I did not own a suit at that time. I felt belittled and embarrassed and tried to find a few suits I could afford at TJ Maxx to wear to practicum. This book described my own internal conflicts perfectly – how could I stay true to my blue-collar roots and values while entering a white-collar professional world? Likewise, would I be truly accepted in either once becoming a doctor? Being aware of, and accepting of, my identity has helped me to consider the experiences and identity of my clients and their families, as well as the systemic challenges they may face.

My private practice serves children and families who are uninsured or those who are receiving Medicaid, and the majority of the families I work with are on restricted incomes. As such, the intersectionality of socioeconomic status with other aspects of identity and culture plays a predominate role in the work that I do. Even though the majority of the clients I work with are Caucasian, I work with many children who are biracial, or of different races than their parents as they are in the foster care system or have been adopted. This presents some challenges for many of the children I work with, as there is not a lot of diversity within the community or schools.

Clair Mellenthin, MSW, RPT-S

Issues of intersectionality are important to recognize in play therapy practice. While it is easy to observe the overt gender, racial, or ethnic characteristics and makeup of a person, the more "invisible" or less overt issues such as class, religion, sexuality, and socioeconomic status that are intertwined to create the intersectionality of how different systems of oppression and discrimination impact the client and their family may be less easily identified. Wilson, White, Jefferson, and Danis (2019) stated, "An intersectional conceptual framework also requires an exploration of how institutional practices within the clinical environment, even those that seem neutral, unfairly advantage some and disadvantage others" (p.9). This can be uncomfortable for many therapists to consider, and ask yourself, "Does my clinical practice do this unintentionally?"

As a social worker and play therapist, this has been something I have grappled with over the years. The agency I work at tends to cater toward the middle-upper class, whose families can afford to pay for private therapy sessions and have the financial resources to seek out help as needed. Although we offer very reduced costs to work with the graduate interns, the cost of therapeutic services may shut out those who cannot afford to pay for these services. Other areas of oppression and discrimination occur more broadly in the community, as overall, the city where I reside, and work is ethnically and culturally highly heterogeneous. The majority of the community members attend and are members of a dominant religious organization. For those who are not a part of the ethnic or religious majority, intentional and unintentional discrimination occurs on a regular, consistent basis.

As a play therapist, it is important to recognize these outside cultural factors occurring in the community and how this shapes my client's, as well as my own, life experience. It is also important to recognize that everyone will have their own individual experience within the confines of these outside forces. It is important to be aware of and recognize microaggressions in the playroom and be aware of your own personal biases. Microaggressions may occur if you are taking over for a child who is capable of completing a specific task such as cutting with scissors, dressing up a doll, or setting up a gender-specific play theme; talking in a certain tone of voice; or minimizing (or maximizing) emotional and/or behavioral challenges of certain clients. Do you have certain expectations of how boys and girls *should* act, let alone a child who identifies as nonbinary or LGBTQIA? Have you asked your client how they feel in their world? Wilson et al., shares a poignant advice: "Rather than pretending that differences do not exist, or minimizing their potential impact on the patient-clinician relationship, intersectionality acknowledges how multifaceted differences shape the patient-clinician interaction and forces a reframing that can lead to improved outcomes" (2019).

I know that when I ask my clients what it feels like to take a walk in their shoes and not assume to know or understand, our clinical work and therapeutic relationship deepens and is enhanced. I believe that we can be the best advocates for our clients in a multitude of systems and become a voice for the voiceless – and our playrooms are the first place to start.

Akiko J. Ohnogi, PsyD

I address issues of intersectionality just as I would anything else. As I have clients who are from different educational backgrounds, countries, and social statuses, and speak different languages, I am therefore prescriptive with how I theorize each case, assess what would be most effective for them, and what interventions I utilize. Depending on the client's race, gender, sexuality, and class, I consider both the type of systemic oppression and discrimination that the client has experienced, as well as their reported individual experiences.

I was raised in a nontypical upbringing for a Japanese national (which has led to very different life experiences than the average Japanese middle-class female). My basic assumption is that everyone has had a unique life experience that has affected who they are. Along with this, their various cultural aspects (e.g., race, gender, sexuality, and class) are further contributors to what they experience. I always ask for specific information about various aspects of each client's life, continually keeping an open mind as to what the individual client's experiences have been, including specific systemic oppression and discrimination. I do not make assumptions of the client in front of me based on their social identity, nor ignore the fact that issues of intersectionality may, indeed, be experienced by the client.

Apart from the trauma survivor support that I do, my private practice is self-pay (as insurance does not cover mental health in Japan, unless it is for psychotropic medication, or the treatment is conducted at a government-run clinic). Due to this, there is not a wide range of current socioeconomic differences in my clientele. However, their socioeconomic status from their past may vary widely, and they may have had various experiences and perspectives of social roles and economic comfort. As far as race, gender, and sexuality is concerned, clients come from a wide range of backgrounds. I am constantly updating my knowledge as to what a "typical" experience would be for a client with a specific social identity and comparing it with the specific experiences that the client is having.

Mary Anne Peabody, EdD, RPT-S

Trained as a social worker, I believe race, gender, and other systems of inequality converge and interact. I also believe oppression, discrimination, and privilege are ever present occurring simultaneously at individual, cultural, and institutional levels (family, school, community, society). From this multilevel stance, I am aware we live in a highly stratified society, where categories or primary statuses exist. I too am situated in this web of interacting identities due to my own categories or primary statuses. I am affected by and benefit from existing social systems where inequality is present, so naturally my child clients and their parents/caregivers are also undoubtedly affected by intersecting axes of inequality.

As a therapist, my clients present with these interacting identities and often with complex backgrounds. My goals for clients align with generalist goals of social work practice and typically include enhancing peoples coping and problem-solving capacities, creating opportunities for empowerment, linking people with resources and services, and if necessary, advocating for social policy or practice improvement (Cox et al., 2019). Therefore, my individual actions as a therapist and my standards of practice as a social worker are to treat humans with respect and to continue to be an ally by taking personal responsibility to facilitate empowerment in others.

Along this journey, I have made and continue to make my fair share of mistakes and I try to learn from my mistakes. I work hard to be aware of my own biases and address these issues by staying current in the literature from not only my primary field of social work but other interdisciplinary readings. I have worked in public contexts most of my career, including public schools and now a public state university. The latter offers me a very valuable perspective, especially among a disparate student population where some students experience multiplicative disadvantages while others experience multiplicative advantages (King, 1988).

I am fortunate to teach in a department at the university that offers an interdisciplinary major. Accordingly, my closest colleagues are professors from the fields of women and gender studies, psychology, social work, sociology, anthropology, and leadership. Our university consistently offers professional development opportunities, study groups, and student-led dialogues on social justice issues including topics of intersectionality. By the very fact that I am privileged to have had access to higher education, I believe I should use this privilege to help others. As a professor and practitioner-scholar, I am part of a circle of influence for a new generation of students. I take this as the highest honor.

Finally, as a prescriptive play therapist I always challenge one-size-fits-all models in therapy (Kaduson et al., 2020) and extend this challenge to the topic of intersectionality. We must, as child and family therapists, be aware of the intersectionality-informed issues facing the children and families we serve in play therapy. There is no one-size-fits-all model of play therapy and no one-size-fits-all way of thinking about children and families.

Dee Ray, PhD, RPT-S

The playroom is a place of acceptance, a place in which the environment (i.e., the therapist, the room, and the materials) is constructed to send messages of unconditional positive regard to the child at all times. Unconditional positive regard involves the therapist's warm acceptance of the child but, beyond acceptance, unconditional positive regard is an experience of prizing the child. The play therapist prizes the child holistically and the experience of being with the child. All identities and expressions of identity are valued by the play therapist as vital to understanding the world of the child. Materials in the playroom are carefully selected to allow for expression and exploration of race, gender, sexuality, ability, and status. Children are provided with the symbolic means to address the complicated experiences of growing up in a world where their identities may conflict with the values of their families or communities. My role as the play therapist is to facilitate an environment and relationship in which the child feels free to engage in exploration of identities that may be confusing for the child. Typical child development encompasses the child's movement toward building self-concept, a structure of self within the child's community and greater world. Healthy self-concept is built through the integration of the child's multiple identities which is a process of discovery for each child. In child-centered play therapy, the process of self-discovery is supported through a focus on child-directed play and relational support during times of discovery.

Systemically, I address issues of intersectionality through parent and community education. Although I believe that my essential role with the child is to support the child's self-direction, my essential role with systemic partners is to facilitate their abilities to provide an accepting environment for the child. My role is often to educate parents, caretakers, school staff, and other adults in the child's life regarding the nature and effects of growing up in a system in which a child feels misunderstood, powerless, and unacceptable. Open communication about issues of race, sexuality, economic status, gender identity, religion, and culture is critical to working with parents and children in a way in which both feel encouraged. I broach sensitive subjects by asking parents about their values, their culture, and how those fit with their parenting style and their relationship with their child. My acceptance of the parent's values serves as the basis for the parent to provide acceptance for their child. Just as in play therapy, as the parent feels understood and accepted, they are free to provide acceptance and understanding for their child.

Jessica Stone, PhD, RPT-S

Intersectionality is a term that works to move past the mutually exclusive concepts of race, class, or other socially defined groupings. Kimberlé Crenshaw created this term 30 years ago to explain the oppression of African American women. Since that time the definition and use has broadened. Now, according to Crenshaw,

> Intersectionality is a lens through which you can see where power comes and collides, where it interlocks and intersects. It's not simply that there's a race problem here, a gender problem here, and a class or LBGTQ problem there. Many times that framework erases what happens to people who are subject to all of these things.
>
> (Columbia, 2017)

These intersections of society's groupings, the assumptions made about and within them, the treatment of those within the groupings, and the internal experience of those effected are all concepts about which mental health professionals must be aware. Play therapists have an ethical responsibility to achieve, cultivate, and maintain competency, capability, and cultural respect. These concepts are fundamental in my work and I consider them to be critical aspects of my personal and professional integrity.

I have a complicated relationship with grouping people. Humans tend toward this as a way to organize, conceptualize, discuss, and so on. We also group clients in many ways, most prominently, through the process of diagnostic labels. However, the statement "If you have met one person with x, then you have met one person" blares loudly in my head. It then becomes critical to understand labels and groupings for the limited uses they have, be aware of any intersectionality and the effects as much as possible, and see our clients for who that person is and what s/he brings into the room.

Overall, a play therapist should have the foci of meeting the client where they are understanding their needs and goals, and recognize why they are in the treatment – to have relief in their life in one or more areas. The play therapist has an ethical and professional responsibility to expand his/her own knowledge, to understand that clients can be affected by multiple internal and external effects, to be self-aware of one's own limitations, and to be able to acknowledge and identify if a client triggers responses within the therapist. If such responses are triggered, supervision, guidance, consultation, and self-exploration should be sought. If the responses are deemed to be detrimental to the client and the therapeutic process, appropriate referrals would need to be given.

Daniel Sweeney, PhD, RPT-S

As a male educator and psychotherapist, with considerable recognized and unrecognized privilege, it is my responsibility to be on a lifelong journey of exploration, awareness, and action in regard to issues of intersectionality. There are multiple definitions of intersectionality, but for this question's response, I will use a relatively short and straightforward one: Davis (2008) defines intersectionality as "the interaction between gender, race, and other categories of difference in individual lives, social practices, institutional arrangements, and cultural ideologies and the outcomes of these interactions in terms of power" (p. 68).

I am not sure that the play therapy world is any more enlightened on issues of diversity and intersectionality than any other mental health area. In survey responses including APT members, Penn and Post (2012) report that the demographics included 87.5% Caucasian and 91.8% female. They reported that play therapists "with higher multicultural counseling competence had a greater awareness of White people's racial privilege, institutional discrimination, and blatant racial issues in society" (p. 25). Yet, 31.1% reported having only one multicultural counseling course, and 37.7% reported having between 0 and 6 hours of multiculturally related CE (2012).

Unfortunately, as noted by Yousef and Ener (2014), the "recent trend of multicultural implications in the counseling profession and work with children has not significantly translated into play therapy research" (p. 95). They also note that the "knowledge, skills, and instructional methods related to ensuring play therapists are trained in multicultural competencies remains abstract" (p. 98).

It is my responsibility to have as a playroom that is equipped with culturally diverse toys and gender fluid dolls/puppets. It is important that my playroom, while being well-equipped and care for, does not have an appearance of being a high SES type of environment. It is important that I take my time to be sensitive and understand of issues of marginalization and privilege with my child clients and their parents. I have made referrals to play therapists of color and nonmale play therapists, when this has been the preference of both current and prospective clients. I am open to and appreciative of feedback from colleagues, when my own privilege has blurred my awareness to marginalized populations. It is a journey that I hope to always engage and travel on.

References

Ansbacher, H., & Ansbacher, R. (Eds.). (1956). *The individual psychology of Alfred Adler: A systematic presentation in selections from his writings.* Harper and Row.

Carlson, J., Watts, R., & Maniacci, M. (2005). *Adlerian therapy: Theory and practice.* American Psychological Association.

Columbia (2017, June 8). *Kimberlé Crenshaw on intersectionality, more than two decades later.* https://www.law.columbia.edu/pt-br/news/2017/06/kimberle-crenshaw-intersectionality.

Cox, L. E., Tice, C. J., & Long, D. D. (2019). *Introduction to social work* (2nd ed.). Sage.

Crenshaw, K. (1989). Demarginalizing the intersection of race and sex: A black feminist critique of antidiscrimination doctrine, feminist theory and antiracist politics. *The University of Chicago Legal Forum, 1,* 139–167.

Davis, K. (2008). Intersectionality as buzzword: A sociology of science perspective on what makes a feminist theory successful. *Feminist Theory, 9,* 67–85.

Drewes, A. A. (2005). Play in selected cultures: Diversity and universality. In E. Gil & A. A. Drewes (Eds.), *Cultural issues in play therapy* (pp. 26–71). Guilford Press.

Grzanka, P. R., Santos, C. E., & Moradi, B. (2017). Intersectionality research in counseling psychology. *Journal of Counseling Psychology, 64,* 453–457.

Hancock, A. M. (2016). *Intersectionality: An intellectual history.* Oxford University Press.

Herring, R., & Runion, K. (1994). Counseling ethnic children and youth from an Adlerian perspective. *Journal of Multicultural Counseling and Development, 22,* 215–226.

Moradi, B., & Grzanka, P. R. (2017). Using intersectionality responsibly: Toward critical epistemology, structural analysis, and social justice activism. *Journal of Counseling Psychology, 64,* 500–513.

Kaduson, H. G., Cangelosi, D., & Schaefer, C. E. (2020) *Prescriptive play therapy* (p. ix). Guilford.

King, D. K. (1988). Multiple jeopardy, multiple consciousness: The context of a black feminist ideology. *Signs: Journal of Women in Culture and Society, 14*(1) 42–72.

Lubrano, A. (2005). *Limbo: Blue-collar roots, white-collar dreams.* Wiley Press.

Penn, S., & Post, P. (2012). Investigating various dimensions of play therapists' self-reported multicultural counseling competence. *International Journal of Play Therapy, 21*(1), 14–29.

Wilson, Y., White, A., Jefferson, A., & Danis, M. (2019). Intersectionality in clinical medicine: The need for a conceptual framework. *The American Journal of Bioethics, 19*(2), 8–19.

Yousef, D., & Ener, L. (2014). Multicultural considerations in graduate play therapy courses. *International Journal of Play Therapy, 23*(2), 90–99.

Part III

Practice

15 What Are Your Suggestions for Building a Successful Play Therapy Practice?

Jeff Ashby, PhD, RPT-S

My suggestions for building a successful play therapy practice fall into two primary categories. First, get better at the practice of play therapy. The systematic development of your therapeutic skills in the application of play therapy is the best way to build a successful play therapy practice. The really good play therapists I know in private practice are all full, with a wait list. They will take my referrals as a favor (and because they are gracious and lovely people), but not because they have openings in their caseload. They are really good play therapists and, as a result, have successful practices. It isn't an accident that these really good play therapists, with very successful play therapy practices, are all RPTs and regularly engage in professional consultation. They have engaged in the systematic program of developing expertise in play therapy organized in the registry of play therapists administered by the Association of Play Therapy. This system offers a deliberate and intentional path to develop play therapy expertise and be recognized for the same. In addition, the successful play therapists I know all regularly engage in peer consultation because they are interested in continuing to grow in their play therapy skills.

The second suggestion I would make to develop a successful play therapy practice is to build your business skills. Especially if you are in private practice, or planning to move into private practice, it is essential to build your business skills. There are lots of really gifted therapists who have been unsuccessful in building a practice because they did not have the necessary business skills. It sometimes feels like a paradigm shift but, if you are starting a private practice, you are launching a business. You need a business plan, legal advice, accounting, bookkeeping, and billing services. It takes two different skill sets to, on the one hand, be a good therapist and, on the other hand, run a successful business. A successful play therapy practice requires both sets of skills. The good news is that many business skills and services can be outsourced. You can hire great people to help you develop a business plan and manage budgets, and so on. However, you need to realize that you need these skills. I would argue that "if you build it they will come" might work in the movies (Robinson, 1989) but won't work if you're trying to build a successful play therapy practice.

Robert Jason Grant, EdD, RPT-S

Success can be defined many ways. I don't believe successful means quantity as in how large or how many practices a person manages, but it is more about the quality of the work being performed and personal fulfillment and satisfaction that a therapist feels. Most play therapists are not business oriented yet find themselves in situations where they are operating a business. The combination of feeling purposeful in the work the therapist is doing and pragmatically operating a business can be a challenging combination. I have been fortunate to own and operate a private practice clinic for many years and have had great success by any definition. Based on this, I would suggest a successful play therapy practice might possess the following.

1   The therapist has a thorough understanding of play therapy theories and approaches, and understands child growth and development.
2   The play therapist possesses an understanding of how to engage with and work with parents and families, not just the individual child.
3   The play therapist is knowledgeable in setting up a playroom or play space in which to provide therapy for children. This would include understanding how to set up a playroom based on play therapy theory and selecting appropriate toys and materials for the clientele the therapist will be seeing.
4   The play therapist has accountability and consultation opportunities established with other play therapists. There is a continuous ability to acquire feedback and be monitored to ensure the play therapist is providing appropriate therapy and management of his or her practice.
5   The play therapist is connected with a play therapy organization.
6   The play therapist participates in continuing education to maintain learning and growth about play therapy.
7   The play therapist is aware of best practices in his or her discipline and strives to abide by and perform best practices guidelines. This would include conducting himself or herself professionally and abiding by ethical guidelines.
8   Being able to explain, educate about, and promote play therapy.
9   Effectively marketing the play therapy practice in the therapist's local community.
10 Understanding the basics of operating a business – the pragmatics of business management and legal issues.

Heidi Gerard Kaduson, PhD, RPT-S

First and foremost, before starting a practice you must become licensed as a mental health professional (or school-based counselor) and make sure you have had a lot of training and supervision from Registered Play Therapist-Supervisors so that when you are with a child, your technical brain is at rest and you are focused totally on the client. There is so much new information through research and clinical practice that will influence how and when you interact with a child. I believe in being open to any and everything that can enhance my knowledge of what best suits a child's ability to self-heal. Child therapists, especially well-trained play therapists, are needed more than ever before. We must be open to learning more and teaching more whenever possible. I truly believe that educating teachers, parents, and colleagues about play therapy also will expand anyone's practice. Go to Parent-Teacher Organization meetings, conferences, and so on, and share your knowledge. Keeping a network available to bounce off questions and comments will assist in allowing the therapist to have supervision available.

The therapist must know all stages of child development and be willing to assist in the child's life outside of the practice (school, home, etc.). Continue to learn and keep a realistic expectation of helping one child. Then, when you are truly genuine and present with the client, you will see the expansion of the practice develop. I believe that the key to becoming a good play therapist with a successful play therapy practice is being playful to illicit the therapeutic powers of play. On a completely different level, play therapists have to be realistic about how much one can do for any one child. There are limits set by money, schools, laws, and so on. In order to have a thriving practice, you must really believe in the therapeutic powers of play, as well as the fact that children can heal themselves in a safe playroom with a genuine play therapist. You also need a high tolerance for messiness because I believe that no child should have to clean after themselves in play therapy. In addition, you really need to be able to trust the process and respect the roles of parents and caregivers in a child's life. Many of them need support as well. While you certainly need to give control over to the child in the playroom, you must become comfortable with that and trust that a child will guide you where they need to go. Furthermore, if you are in an area of few or no play therapists, it will increase your demand, and you will become the expert in that area in your town. Maintaining a busy practice has always been part of my way of treating children, and word of mouth will get you a thriving practice.

Jennifer Lefebre, PsyD, RPT-S

Create a solid business plan. It doesn't need to be formal; it should just cover where you see yourself in six months, one year, three years, five years, and so on. The plan should look at case load, finances, professional development, space – all aspects – and should start small. An important piece of this is also defining your specialty area and the market around where you want to practice. I started out my private practice by renting a small room in a friend's office. I then rented what affectionately became known as "the therapy shack", which was a bright yellow and blue renovated two car garage. It had a tiny waiting room and a wood stove for heat – I had a toilet and sink in a closet for a rest room! I then moved into a store front, and now I am in a small building that has four office rooms, a training space, and a large waiting room. My next plan is opening a full-fledged trauma center in an old Victorian house.

A vital step to having a successful play therapy practice is to have a network of colleagues and friends that are passionate about play therapy. We cannot do this work in isolation, and in order to have a successful practice you need people that you can connect with that support you. This can be done in person or virtually. The Association for Play Therapy's local branches are great for getting to know people and there are several groups on social media that support connections between play therapists.

As my career continues to expand in the play therapy and trauma world, I wouldn't be able to do what I do without the love and support of my family and friends. My husband Derek has encouraged me in these recent years to grow my passion for play therapy training, writing, and supervision. My children do the same. I wouldn't be where I am today without their support, love, and encouragement.

Clair Mellenthin, MSW, RPT-S

My top three suggestions for building a successful play therapy practice are first to become credentialed as a Registered Play Therapist (RPT). This credential signifies that you have had extensive training in play therapy practice, theory, and clinical skills building. It also sets you apart from other generalized mental health practitioners so you can speak with authority and demonstrate not only confidence but clinical competence in a specialty practice area. Having the RPT credential has opened up more doors than I ever imagined it would for me professionally, and is one of the reasons I was originally sought out for a television segment that has blossomed into a year-running monthly TV segment on a local television channel.

My next suggestion is to develop a web presence. In today's world, it is important to not only have a user-friendly website for your practice but to also be involved on social media, writing blog posts, speaking on podcasts, and doing other media work. The more your name positively pops up in Google searches, the more clientele will come to your practice. If you are uncomfortable or unfamiliar with technology and media exposure, I would recommend consulting with a media specialist who is knowledgeable and can connect you to different media resources in your area. I would also join an online referral service such as Psychology Today. Many consumers find all of their professional needs and referrals online and rely on online advertising as well as reviews when seeking out a health care provider, and mental health is no different.

My last suggestion is to identify who you really want to work with and develop your passions into a niche that sets you apart from other mental health clinicians in your area. Is there a particular population you are passionate about helping? Is there a specific age group you absolutely love to work with? Speaking at local events, offering your time and services to schools, hospitals, community organizations, and networking groups are also important ways to let people know you exist and to shine a light onto the services you offer, as well as your area of expertise. Some therapists worry that if they narrow their scope of practice, they will limit the number of clients who reach out to them for services. In my experience, your expertise and defined scope of practice helps to set you apart from others and in no way diminishes your marketability or approachability.

Akiko J. Ohnogi, PsyD

People define "successful" differently (financial wealth, full termination of cases, social recognition, etc.). The following suggestions for building a successful play therapy practice are based on my belief that having a practice in which a play therapist feels comfortable and happy defines "successful". Much of this comfort and happiness involves knowing who you want to be as a therapist and what types of clients you want to serve.

Part of being happy with your practice is having one. It's important to make sure that people in your community are aware of your existence to the extent that you have enough exposure and feel comfortable. This can be done in various ways, whether it be to advertise, socialize, volunteer, provide workshops, and so on. In my case, I do not advertise, as most of my clients come by word of mouth. They are referred by current and former clients, schools, mental health practitioners, other professionals (medical practitioners, lawyers), embassies, and so on. This is a result of attending conferences and professional gatherings around that provide potential referral sources. I also facilitate workshops at various schools, companies, institutions, and so on, and this helps others learn about my practice.

As a part of choosing where to get exposure, it is important that you know your potential clientele pool. A play therapist should be knowledgeable of where the specific types of clients they desire are located. Advertising and socializing will be more effective if your information is reaching the types of clients who need the services you are providing.

It is also important to be clear within yourself regarding the issues and age ranges that you would like to provide services to. Consider if you would like to specialize in one or multiple issues or be a general practitioner? I see a wide range of clients (age, issues, referral sources, and culture), and I am known to specialize in working with trauma survivors of natural disasters, multicultural families, and young children. Developing the type of therapist you want to be and the type of practice you want to operate with can be a significant part of feeling successful.

Mary Anne Peabody, EdD, RPT-S

To build a successful play therapy practice requires focused attention on your referral sources. I believe focused attention of building collaborations with pediatricians and family practice physicians should be top priority. My biggest referral sources in private practice were several local pediatricians and family practice physicians who had established long and trusted relationships with parents. When the physician would recommend me as a therapist for their child, it seemed to add an additional layer of credibility. Valuing this collaboration, I continuously made efforts to keep my name and practice in the forefront of these physicians. I sent several of the Association of Play Therapy's pediatrician brochure to their offices available through the store function on the APT website: www.a4pt.org and included my business cards.

Likewise, I made strong efforts to consult with area school counselors, social workers, and school psychologists as another tier of potential referrals. After many years in the school setting, I discovered my years in private practice to be isolating. To balance this, I intentionally sought out group consultation opportunities to build networking and to continue my professional development. This was a professional gift to myself and simultaneously built collaborative relationships that in turn translated into many more referrals over the years.

I would also suggest taking opportunities to be a guest speaker in local university social work, counseling, or psychology courses and be willing to speak at school counselor annual conferences. Additionally, exhibiting at the statewide conferences offers unique opportunities for one-to-one conversations. Like any business, taking time to market and nurture referral sources is time well spent.

Dee Ray, PhD, RPT-S

Throughout my career, I have worked in nonprofit settings providing play therapy to children of families who operate with limited financial resources. My concept of a successful practice is reaching children whose families are not initially aware of services, wary of such services, or do not have the financial means to pay for services. My suggestions are given within this scope of practice. My first suggestion is that successful practice is predicated on the competence and knowledge of the play therapist. The play therapist is knowledgeable of information that affects practice, including child development, current child trends, and play therapy, among a substantial amount of other relevant information necessary for competent practice. The play therapist is well-trained and skillful in the provision of play therapy as evidenced through staying current in education and consultation.

Second, the play therapist who manages a successful practice for children in nonprofit settings works within a social justice framework in which the therapist operates from high levels of awareness of privilege while attempting to advocate and meet the needs of underserved populations. Structural systems of care including marketing, paperwork, initial contact, scheduling, and language are designed to be sensitive to populations who may have limited education, resources, or systemic power. When play therapists are sensitive to these dynamics, families are more likely to seek services for their children.

A third practical suggestion is the importance of administrative organizational abilities. My experience is that most play therapists like to help people through providing services of care directly to children and families. Play therapists often tend to dislike the organizational components of practice such as treatment planning, case notes, and formal evaluation of services. However, these organizational processes are critical to the success of a practice. I encourage play therapists to set aside time each day to attend to these less immediately rewarding activities because they often end up being stumbling blocks to play therapists down the road when they have procrastinated the performance of these duties.

Jessica Stone, PhD, RPT-S

A key component of this question is for the play therapist to define what success means to him or her. Some primary areas include: financial, professional, personal, academic, and clinical. Thinking through what success means for one's self can greatly inform the direction and trajectory of the play therapy practice.

Financial success can be thought of in terms of short- and long-term goals. If one has those goals defined, then decisions about things such as the number of clients needed per week can be determined. These would potentially change over time with the ebb and flow of life phases. Is there a desired annual increase? How are hourly rates determined? Is it more beneficial to work for an agency or environment (school, hospital, etc.)? Or is it better to risk the variability of a private setting?

Professional success can include topics such as position within the community, participation in a variety of field-related roles (serving on a professional committee, etc.), presenting at conferences, writing, or even implementing new ideas or services. What is important to achieve with regards to professional success?

What are the important personal successes one would like to realize? Personal goals can include learning new skills, focusing on self-care, relationship goals, family, travel, bucket list items, and so on. How do these personal successes complement the professional goals?

Some practitioners would like to attain a certain level of academic success. This could include pursuing a higher degree or specialty. This can also include teaching and other roles within academia. This category also includes writing and presenting.

What kind of clinical goals are important? Would you like to achieve a word-of-mouth referral-based practice? Would you like to receive training, experience, and supervision to specialize in a certain area? Would you like to achieve a particular level of satisfied clients and, if so, how would you determine the satisfaction levels? Would you like to achieve client success, local community success, or success in a certain field or perhaps all three? How would these goals be realized?

The definition of success will vary from person to person and must be defined within each individual. It can also develop and change over time. For me, I strive for success in all of these areas. I want to work smarter and reach some financial goals with the client load I carry. I pay attention to local pay scales and determine my per session rate based on a formula of the current going rate combined with what I believe my specific treatment is worth. I have entered a phase of industry (creating new concepts and products for use within therapy treatment), writing, mentoring, supervising, teaching, and presenting. I have served on boards and committees to give back to my professional community and contribute what I have learned in almost three decades of this work. I look for life and work balance so that I can enjoy my family, experience "downtime", and continue the work. I aspire to be thought of as someone who loved the work, to learn, to share, and to be involved, and worked hard to be the best provider I can be for my clients. This is what success looks like for me. What does it look like for you?

Daniel Sweeney, PhD, RPT-S

Of all of the questions in this chapter, this is the one that I have the least on which to comment. I have never had a full-time private practice, in play therapy, or in general psychotherapy. I have always worked for an agency, organization, or university – on a full-time basis. All of the private practice that I have done has been done on a part-time basis.

When I started my career, the advice would be to have thousands of business cards and do a lot of face-to-face networking. This can still be helpful. However, what is more important is to develop contacts electronically through the creation and maintenance of a strong web presence and social media network (Meyers, 2019). As play therapists, maintaining a strong relationship and presence with the APT – nationally, as well as state branches and local branches – is very important. This includes giving presentations at all of these levels.

Part of having an internet presence is having an attractive and easy-to-navigate website. Pictures of any therapists and playroom(s) at the private practice should be included. A short video is always helpful to explain what play therapy is and how it is successful. Most therapists (and play therapists!) enter the field with a focus on providing a quality service, which is important. However, being skilled as a business and marketing person is as important in terms of building and maintaining a private practice.

References

Meyers, L. (2019). Establishing a private practice. *Counseling Today*. https://ct.counseling.org/2019/03/establishing-a-private-practice.

Robinson, P. A. (Director). (1989). *Field of dreams* (Film). Universal Pictures.

16 What Do You Think Is One of the Most Challenging Ethical Issues Currently in Play Therapy?

Jeff Ashby, PhD, RPT-S

I think one of the most challenging ethical issues currently in play therapy is the use of technology in communication with clients and in storing client information. Confidentiality is a fundamental maxim of ethical therapy identified and discussed in all of the major mental health ethical codes (e.g., ACA, 2014; APA, 2010; NASW, 2017) as well as the practice guidelines for play therapy (APT, 2009). The current challenge for play therapists is to protect confidentiality in this digital age. Electronic mail, text messaging, electronic medical records, electronically processed credit card payments, the Internet, and social media are prominent in the practices of most play therapists and few of us have considered the intricacies of how to maintain confidentiality in these various platforms and processes. In addition, the Health Insurance Portability and Accountability Act (HIPAA) provides a legal mandate for specific protection of client information. Finally, keeping up with technology is a "moving target" as the rate of technological change is exponential.

While there are some helpful references to help play therapists consider the legal and ethical risks of technology in practice (Lustgarten & Elhai, 2018), a few simple suggestions have helped me. First, review your codes and the law. As much as many of us reference the ethical codes and pertinent law (e.g., HIPAA), some of us (okay, me) are less likely to actually look at exactly what the codes say. Several of the codes (e.g., ACA, NASW) have more recently updated sections that do speak to issues of technology. In addition, there are sections of HIPAA that can help us navigate these issues (e.g., understanding the importance of securing Business Associate Agreements with technology entities). Second, review and update your informed consent (Barnett, 2018). No matter where you come down on issues like electronic mail and texting, having a clear informed consent, including sections on social media, is extremely helpful and helps you start an open dialogue with clients about expectations and boundaries (Kolmes, 2012).

Robert Jason Grant, EdD, RPT-S

Ethical dilemmas can manifest at any time. Many of them are small in scale and specific to an individual situation. I have witnessed some ethical issues that many play therapists appear to be navigating on a regular basis. One issue being the popularity and usage of social media and technology. There seems to be a lot more questions than answers when it comes to how a play therapists and other mental health providers utilize, engage with, and navigate social media and the Internet. I have spent a fair amount of time talking to my licensing board, reviewing best practices and ethical guidelines of national mental health organizations, and conversing with peers on how to utilize social media and what to avoid from a business perspective.

Unfortunately, there has not always been a clear guide or consensus. There seems to be a clear understanding that therapists should not be "friends" with a client on a personal social media account but "business" accounts are something that clients can like and follow. It is fairly well established that therapists should not discuss clients through a social media outlet nor interact with clients on social media. However, much of this is new territory and is still being conceptualized in terms of best practices and ethics. It might seem easier to abandon the whole arena of social media, but these platforms are providing some promising and helpful opportunities for therapists to market, promote, and provide resources. How to utilize the benefits and avoid unethical practices is certainly one of the things I see as current ethical issue for play therapists.

Another issue, which is specific to play therapy, is the misuse and misrepresentation of play therapy. The Association for Play Therapy works diligently to provide accurate and accessible information about what play therapy is and is not. The organization publishes promotional and educational material and encourages the pursuit of Registered Play Therapist (RPT), Registered Play Therapist-Supervisor (RPT-S), and School Based-Registered Play Therapist (SB-RPT) credentials to ensure someone has appropriate knowledge of play therapy. Unfortunately, there are many professionals in the mental health field and sometimes outside of the mental health field who call themselves play therapists or say they are implementing play therapy, but they are inaccurate, misleading, and unknowledgeable about play therapy. They are not really implementing play therapy, and this causes confusion in the client community and serious misunderstandings about what play therapy is and how it can help a child and family.

I try to address misrepresentation in my local community by engaging in speaking events about play therapy, periodically posting about play therapy in my business social media accounts and distributing play therapy brochures. For play therapists, this is an ongoing ethical issue which is a struggle to resolve. For now, the best course of action I have found is to be very public in educating about and promoting play therapy in an accurate and clear manner.

Heidi Gerard Kaduson, PhD, RPT-S

Since children process their psychological difficulties through play, and play is nonliteral, it is often a challenge to decide how much of the play should be shared in progress notes or with caregivers. I believe the most challenging ethical issues come when trying to work within ethical frameworks, dealing with conflict between parties, and managing safeguarding issues (Jackson, 1998). All mental health specialists (counselors, psychologists, psychiatrists, and social workers) are bound by ethical principles of doing no harm, which helps mitigate the problems of inadequate training, but not all understand what this means when it comes to play therapy. Children heal themselves within a safe play therapy room, a well-trained play therapist, and through the therapeutic powers of play. We must keep or contain the play as children process their difficulties. When there is a chance of sabotage by caregivers or misunderstanding about the play itself by them, we must balance what is needed to be ethically bound by informed consent and confidentiality. As play therapists, we have an ethical responsibility for accountability to our clients. But who is the client? In many cases, it is the caregiver. When we find the caregiver not capable or willing to work in the best interests of the child, we must consider how we can assist the child and/or caregiver to allow for needed changes.

It is very important as play therapists to understand the therapeutic powers of play and remember that play is nonliteral. Therefore, although the therapeutic powers of play are always at work, what you believe you are witnessing in children's play may not be correct. It is very important to follow the lead of the child, but do not overgeneralize information you see in the play. Explore more to find out whether the child is at risk or has been coached to say or do certain things. Whatever course we take in play therapy (with the child, caregiver, and/or family), it is important to use interventions for which there is empirical support. Each case can be completely different in its presentation. Keeping the child in a place that does no harm is of utmost importance, and so the communication between therapists and caregivers can be ethically challenging. Supervision should be ongoing even when you are a seasoned play therapist where issues like these can be discussed and processed with the most appropriate outcome.

Jennifer Lefebre, PsyD, RPT-S

I would say confidentiality is a challenging ethical dilemma in working with children, as we are placed in a unique position of holding a child's thoughts and feelings in privacy, while the parent is the true client based on consent. This can become an issue in terms of mandated reporting, child custody, or other legal matters. Additionally, insurance companies, court systems, child welfare, and schools often want things to "have happened yesterday", and are not on the same wavelength of understanding the true process of therapy. This can create ethical issues around record keeping, in terms of who may be requesting records and what they truly need access to.

Practicing in a rural community, the ethical issue of multiple relationships often comes up. I am the only psychologist, and the only registered play therapist, in the county – and I take Medicaid. My options for making referrals to other clinicians is extremely limited, and deciding to live and work in a semirural community (my town has 1,400 people) means that I am likely to have preexisting relationships with some of my clients. In this setting the question is, "How could I engage in a safe, nonexploitative multiple relationship?"

I have worked with children that attend school and play sports with my children, and as I volunteer at many of these activities, I am placed in a dual role. I have served nachos and ice cream to some of my clients at football games, and I often see families while shopping or out with my family. I let families know that there is a strong possibility that we may cross paths, and if a client indicates that they are currently connected with me in some way (through my children or community), we discuss it and decide the path that is best for the client, and come to an understanding about boundaries and how to manage when our paths cross outside of the play therapy room.

Clair Mellenthin, MSW, RPT-S

I think one of the most challenging ethical issues happening in the field of play therapy has been therapists practicing outside their scope of practice and not receiving adequate in-depth training and play therapy supervision to treat complicated cases and disorders. In the past, you could receive most if not all of your necessary continuing education hours from an online format without ever attending an in-person training. While this use of technology can be helpful and is necessary in today's world, there is no replacement for live in-person training and instruction. My hope is with the new credentialing standards from APT, this problem will decrease with time and with this next generation of play therapists who are coming into this field.

Another ethical issue I find while training play therapists around the globe and in the United States is that there are many therapists that are excited to learn new techniques, and are happy to buy play therapy technique books but lack a clear understanding of theory and the importance of clearly identifying the theoretical underpinning of each play therapy intervention. Without this knowledge and understanding, you are at real risk of causing harm to your clients, as you may not be fully prepared for your client's emotional response or need for containment. You may also be ill-equipped to understand the potential ramifications and consequences that this lack of awareness and understanding can cause in the long term. You have to understand why you are doing what you are doing and be able to articulate the therapeutic rationale for the different theoretical approaches and interventions. Attending a 1–2-day workshop does not qualify you as an expert in a particular treatment approach and I worry that there is a belief and underlying instant-gratification expectation that is permeating our field and newer clinicians.

Lastly, I believe an ethical issue in the field of play therapy is individuals marketing themselves online and in play therapy trainings as specialists in all areas of child and adolescent mental health and play therapy approaches. You can't be an expert in all things. While many clinicians practice as a general practitioner and treat a wide variety of treatment issues, these clinicians function similar to an emergency room (ER) doctor. An ER doctor can present and should present on the issues they treat in the ER, but it would be inappropriate for them to speak about oncology or end-of-life treatment. As a dear friend of mine, who is an ER physician, stated, "I know just enough of everything to be knowledgeable and lack enough knowledge of everything to be dangerous if I am not aware of what I am doing and treating". I think this applies in the field of mental health as well.

Akiko J. Ohnogi, PsyD

I think there are many challenging ethical issues currently in play therapy. Some that I have encountered more recently include when to keep information from a parent based on the child's confidentiality, especially when working with a child who is the middle of an acrimonious divorce child custody case; deciding if and how a child abducted by a parent is to be reunited with said parent; working with clients that have issues in which I do not specialize in treating, but there are no other professionals available to provide treatment; and ending treatment when the client is no longer able to afford to pay although they still need services.

My most challenging ethical issue regards seeing multiple members within a family separately as individual clients due to the lack of qualified and trained mental health professionals available to work with the family. It is my belief that family members who have individual needs for psychological treatment should each have their own mental health clinician. This is to ensure that emotional, psychological, and practical boundaries can be maintained. Emotional triggers (suspicion, jealousy, competitiveness, etc.) that may result from sharing a therapist can be avoided if each person has their own therapist. It also helps ensure confidentiality and avoids potentially awkward situations for the client and therapist.

There are many areas around the world where access to a mental health professional is challenging, and this often occurs in my community. When I decide to see multiple family members as clients, it is extremely important that all the family members are made aware of the risks of being treated by the same clinician. I take care to be especially cognizant of and am prepared to manage the possible emotional effects that seeing more than one family member can have on clients, as well as the conflicts it may create for myself as the therapist. Ethically it is a case-by-case decision based on the circumstances. While it is not always my preferred process (working with multiple family members), in some cases it may be more unethical to deny services that would not otherwise be rendered.

Mary Anne Peabody, EdD, RPT-S

The field of play therapy continues to expand, and access to play therapy information and research is unprecedented. While this explosive growth is exciting, it is not without its ethical challenges. Ethically, play therapists are responsible and accountable to their clients. One aspect of therapist accountability is the responsibility to identify and deliver effective interventions (Bratton & Swan, 2017). Yet this raises several questions. How does the individual play therapist define effective? Is it ethical to use an intervention that has not been studied for effectiveness? Are there differences between the terms empirically supported, empirically informed, evidence-based, and research-based treatments and interventions? These questions and terminology variances can be confusing, conceivably leaving a play therapist to choose interventions or seek professional development training on interventions that have not been proven to be effective. In my opinion, this positions a therapist in an ethical quagmire.

It is well documented that certain treatments are more effective than others for specific disorders (Siev & Chambless, 2007). Additionally, research reviews reporting the empirical base for effective practice of play therapy are readily available to guide therapists in expanding evidence-informed interventions (Baggerly et al., 2010; Reddy et al., 2016) and an evidence-based practice statement to inform therapist clinical decision-making now exists (Ray & McCullough, 2015, revised 2016).

Due to valiant efforts of several play therapy researchers, a number of play therapy treatments now appear on the National Registry of Evidence-Based Programs and Practices (NREPP) provided on the Substance and Mental Health Services Association (SAMHSA) website at https://www.samhsa.gov/ebp-resource-center. Consequently, the sheer number of research studies examining outcome effectiveness continues to grow as evidenced by the creation of an outcome research database found at http://evidencebasedchildtherapy.com/.

In summary, identifying and selecting interventions proven to be effective is no longer a mystery. While current play therapists may be bombarded with copious choices, I believe it is our ethical responsibility to select interventions that have been scientifically proven to be most effective in treating our child clients. Thus, we must remain accountable and responsible to our clients, the field, and ultimately ourselves by continually questioning whether what we just read, studied, or selected as a treatment intervention can pass the ethical litmus test of effectiveness. Our children's mental health is too important to be left to unproven practices and methods.

Dee Ray, PhD, RPT-S

In speaking generally about issues in play therapy, I often feel like a broken record in that I am most concerned about the issue of play therapy training. I think the most challenging ethical issue in the field of play therapy is the competence of play therapists. The continuum of concern ranges from therapists who put board games in their offices and call themselves play therapists without any training at all to credentialed play therapists who randomly engage in techniques based on the latest Internet trend without intentionality or theoretical foundation. There are many well-trained play therapists who practice with integrity. However, I am concerned about the many therapists who provide services to children without proper training in general mental health intervention and/or play therapy. When therapists engage in child therapy without proper and appropriate education and supervision, they may potentially harm children through ineffective and, sometimes, damaging practices.

Associated with concern regarding play therapists' competence is a developing concern regarding play therapists who engage in play therapy with children as a way to work through their own personal mental health issues. I believe that some play therapists who are attracted to working with children are often pursuing meeting their needs through their relationships with children. Some examples include play therapists who have not worked through their own childhood traumas working with children who have experienced trauma, play therapists who have unhealthy and permeable boundaries in their personal lives and extend this to their child clients, or play therapists who have not integrated their personal identities and project these identities onto child clients. Examples of play therapists who use their roles as therapists to work through or neglect their own psychological needs are ubiquitous and disturbing. An essential feature to training and education of play therapists is gatekeeping in order to ensure that therapists are healthy in their approach to facilitating the health of others. Hence, my ethical concerns extend beyond the play therapist to the role of play therapist educators and supervisors in their responsibilities to ensure that play therapists who enter the field engage in self-care that ultimately serves to effectively help clients.

Jessica Stone, PhD, RPT-S

One of the most challenging ethical issues currently in play therapy is determining where the lines are/should be when (1) distinguishing the client's interests, wants, and needs from the therapist's belief system and (2) distinguishing the client's interests, wants, and needs from the family's belief system. I have noticed these concerns when teaching and supervising.

Therapist versus Client

There are certainly obvious and identifiable boundaries regarding a client's interests, wants, and needs, but the more nuanced topics seem to be the less-clear areas. Often therapists refer to their theoretical foundation for guidance regarding how to handle what is brought into the session by the client, but we do not always talk about what to do when difficult or incongruent topics arise. Even determinations based on theory can be difficult to distinguish, that is, is the theory truly understood as a formulation of growth and change (and if so, toward what goal?), or is it a way for the therapist biases, comfort, or convenience to be incorporated (even subconsciously). These are not easy or simple explorations for a therapist to have within themselves, however, they are necessary from time to time to ensure a well thought through approach.

More nuanced topics can include interests, belief systems, opinions, sexual orientation, experiences, and more. Each participant comes into the room with their own – everything. The goal is to have explored one's own beliefs and biases (therapist) so that a determination of therapist-client fit can be made relatively easily. If the therapist's belief system, interests, and so on clash greatly with what the client is bringing into the room, supervision should be sought and/or a referral should be made. The client getting their needs met, within their system, is paramount.

Client versus Family

What if the client's needs are different from the family's? Treatment goals reflecting the family's needs may or may not meet the client's needs. In some situations it is a complicated process to determine what the client's needs are and how to balance them with the system in which they operate.

Avinash de Sousa wrote an article in 2010 discussing ethical issues when working with child and adolescent clients. He stated,

> When a psychiatrist comes face to face with treating a child or an adolescent, the general approach lies in doing what is in the best interest of the child – protecting the privacy of the child's communications, and respecting the child as well as the family regardless of race, religion, socioeconomic status, education, or intellectual level, while promoting and supporting the highest level of development and autonomy for the child. The practice of child and adolescent psychotherapy, in both inpatient and outpatient settings, requires the clinician to establish and maintain rapport with both the patient and his or her parents or guardians.
>
> (de Sousa, 2010, para 3–4)

Even within this important and truthful statement, there can be items to be explored. The key components are best interest of the child, protecting privacy, respecting the child and family regarding race, religion, socioeconomic status, education, intellectual level, and supporting development and autonomy while striving for rapport. There are many areas where each participant's beliefs could create a need for exploration.

What to Do?

A play therapist must balance their own belief systems with those of the child and of the family. When working with minors, the complexity increases for a number of reasons including the addition of a third dynamic – the parents/

family (at times, there are additional systems to include as well). It cannot be assumed that the client, the family, and the therapist hold the same value system, so all three must be accounted for with the following hierarchy: (1) client, (2) parents/family, and (3) therapist. This is not clear cut in terms of practicality. For instance, if the family values differ from the client's and these discrepancies create such significant struggles for the client, a determination of the pros and cons can be explored to determine what serves the client best at the time and in the future. It might serve the client better for the client to adhere to certain familial values until other criteria are met. It is preferable for the client to understand the dynamics of such a decision. If the therapist's values differ from the client's in ways that negatively affect the therapeutic process, the therapist should ethically seek consultation, supervision, training, and/or refer the client elsewhere.

Daniel Sweeney, PhD, RPT-S

There are a number of ethical challenges to consider, but from my perspective, the most challenging ethical issue in the field of play therapy is competence. I have encountered too many clinicians who practice play therapy who are ill-trained and even not trained. I have met "play therapists" who have only read one Virginia Axline book, and I have met play therapists who do not know who Virginia Axline is. I have encountered sand tray therapists who do not know who Dora Kalff is, and I have encountered sand tray therapists who have never had any training. These are probably clinicians who will never read this book.

The Code of Ethics of the American Association for Marriage and Family Therapy (2015) speaks clearly to the issue of competence:

- Marriage and family therapists pursue knowledge of new developments and maintain their competence in marriage and family therapy through education, training, and/or supervised experience. [3.1]
- While developing new skills in specialty areas, marriage and family therapists take steps to ensure the competence of their work and to protect clients from possible harm. [3.6]
- Marriage and family therapists do not diagnose, treat, or advise on problems outside the recognized boundaries of their competencies. [3.10]

The Association for Play Therapy (2019) clearly speaks to competence in their Play Therapy Best Practices:

Play therapists practice only within the scope of their competence. Competence is based on: training, supervised experience, professional credentials (state, national, and international), and professional experience. Play therapists commit to knowledge acquisition and/or skill development pertinent to working with a diverse client population.

(p. 10)

While the APT has the process of becoming credentialed as an RPT (discussed above), I would classify this as fitting in with mandatory ethics, as opposed to aspirational ethics. We should aspire to excellence that are "virtuous" within the realm of competence, ideals that

> underlie the aspirational elements of codes of ethics, that is, virtues point toward ways of being with clients, colleagues, supervisees, or students that go above and beyond minimal or expected ethical obligations. It is the professional counselor's responsibility to advocate for the welfare of clients by becoming informed about both the minimum and aspirational standards of practice.
>
> (Kumpf, 2013, p. 52)

Play therapists obviously need to have a base foundation of knowledge, training, and experience. There are also specialties within the specialty of play therapy. These also require a foundation of knowledge, training, and supervised experience. It's the least we should do for our clients and our field.

References

American Association for Marriage and Family Therapy. (2015). *Code of ethics.* https://www.aamft.org/Legal_Ethics/Code_of_Ethics.aspx.

American Counseling Association (2014). *ACA code of ethics and standards of practice.* Author.

American Psychological Association (2010). *Ethical principles of psychologists and code of conduct.* Author.

Association for Play Therapy (2009). *Play therapy best practices.* Association. https://cdn.ymaws.com/www.a4pt.org/resource/resmgr/publications/best_practices_-_sept_2019.pdf.

Association for Play Therapy (2019). *Play therapy best practices: Clinical, professional & ethical issues.* https://www.a4pt.org/resource/resmgr/publications/best_practices_-_sept_2019.pdf.

Baggerly, J., Ray, D., & Bratton, S. (Eds.). (2010). *Child-centered play therapy research: The evidence for effective practice.* Wiley.

Barnett, J. E. (2018). Integrating technological advances into clinical training and practice: The future is now! *Clinical Psychology Science and Practice, 25*(2), 1–4. https://doi.org/10.1111/cpsp.12233.

Bratton, S., & Swan, A. (2017). Status of play therapy research. In R. L. Steen (Ed.), *Emerging research in play therapy, child counseling and consultation* (pp. 1–19). IGA Global.

De Sousa, A. (2010). Ethical issues in child and adolescent psychiatry: A clinical review. *Indian Journal of Medical Ethics, 7*(3). http://ijme.in/articles/ethical-issues-in-child-and-adolescent-psychotherapy-a-clinical-review/?galley=html#one.

Jackson, Y. (1998). Applying APA ethical guidelines to individual play therapy with children. *International Journal of Play Therapy, 7*(2), 1–15.

Kolmes, K. (2012). Social media: What's your policy? *Good Practice: Tools and Information for Professional Psychologists,* Spring/Summer, 10–18.

Kumpf, C. (2013). Frameworks and models in decision making. In C. Jungers & J. Gregoire (Eds.), *Counseling ethics: Philosophical and professional foundations* (pp. 47–70). Springer Publishing Co.

Lustgarten, S. D., & Elhai, J. D. (2018). Technology use in mental health practice and research: Legal and ethical risks. *Clinical Psychology Science and Practice, 25*(2), 1–10. https://doi.org/10.1111/cpsp.12234.

National Association of Social Workers (NASW) (2017). *Code of ethics.* Author.

Reddy, L. A., Files-Hall, T. M., & Schaefer, C. E. (Eds.). (2016). *Empirically based play interventions for children* (2nd ed.). American Psychological Association.

Ray, D. C., & McCullough, R. (2015, revised 2016). *Evidence-based practice statement: Play therapy* (Research report). http://www.a4pt.org/?page=EvidenceBased.

Siev, J., & Chambless, D. L. (2007). Specificity of treatment effects: Cognitive therapy and relaxation for generalized anxiety and panic disorders. *Journal of Consulting and Clinical Psychology, 75*(4), 513–522.

17 How Do You Set and Maintain Boundaries in the Playroom and with Clients, Parents, Caseworkers, and so on?

Jeff Ashby, Ph.D., RPT-S

The question of boundaries is complex because of the distinctions between practicing in rural vs. urban settings, or in school settings with multiple professionals encountering the play therapy client and parents in differing roles with different obligations. I am fortunate to live in a major metropolitan area and, as a result, keeping firmer boundaries is easier than if I worked and lived in a more rural setting or a smaller city. The most important thing I do to set and maintain appropriate boundaries is to use a detailed informed consent. My informed consent clarifies my role and what clients and their parents can reasonably expect from me. I take care to review sections of the consent verbally with parents before treating the play therapy client. Because I work to make it very clear what the boundaries of the relationship are, it becomes clinically informative when clients push those boundaries. If I have done a good job at informed consent, it is a natural follow-up conversation to have with clients who may be pushing boundaries.

The issue of boundaries is particularly interesting when considering online encounters with clients, parents, caseworkers, and others. Again, setting is important. I am not active on social media and, as a result, have fewer overt encounters and boundaries are easier to define and hold. Play therapists who have a greater online presence on social media and the internet may have more opportunity for boundary pushing. Even if one is not intentionally present in a digital space, the internet has made significant information about play therapists available (e.g., registered political party in voting records, home ownership). As a result, clients may be pushing boundaries by searching for play therapists on the internet and the play therapist may be unaware (Kolmes & Taube, 2016). One of the ways I use to manage digital boundaries is adding a social media policy to my informed consent (Kolmes, 2012). This addition has helped me be intentional in communicating the boundaries of the play therapy relationship and sets expectations for privacy and communication in a digital or electronic space.

Robert Jason Grant, Ed.D., RPT-S

Boundaries with clients and parents begin with the intake session. During the intake process several boundary related issues are covered in print form and verbally explained to both the child and the parents. This would include confidentiality regarding attending therapy and how confidentiality for the child from the parent will be handled. Also included is an explanation that I do not accept gifts, how they can communicate with me between sessions, and that I will not acknowledge them outside of therapy (in public) unless they acknowledge me first. I also have a social media and electronic communication policy form that is given in the intake session which explains how I will and will not interact through social media and electronic methods.

Because I work mostly with children with autism and developmental disorders, I keep the play session very routine and consistent. We typically establish a routine with the first session, and we maintain the routine. It is helpful and regulating for children with development disorders to have consistency and know what to expect. I consider this a boundary as we do not deviate from our routine unless there is a serious reason we need to change something. For example, if we establish that I will check in with the parents first when the family arrives for their appointment and then I will meet with the child, we stay with this routine, it doesn't change session to session unless there is a crisis or very important reason we have to shift the routine.

I often utilize the structuring skill found in filial therapy (VanFleet, 2014) to begin and end the session and manage any disruptions like a bathroom break. I also make sure that sessions start on time and end on time. This is another consistency piece that helps the child with a developmental disorder. They can become very dysregulated waiting in the lobby when it is past their session time. I would consider these things as mutual boundaries for both the client and the therapist. During the session I utilize various limit setting models that can be found in almost any play therapy theory or approach. This would include child-centered play therapy (Landreth, 1991), filial therapy (VanFleet, 2014), and Adlerian play therapy (Kottman & Meany-Walen, 2016).

Most often I use the AutPlay therapy (Grant, 2017) limit setting model because I work predominantly with children with autism and this model was designed to address limits with this population. I try to keep limit setting to a minimal but inevitably limits will have to be set when working with children and I have found the limit setting models in play therapy to be very effective. Maintaining boundaries with other professionals who might be involved with the child or family such as a caseworker, an attorney, or an in-home aide can be a little more challenging. I try to keep interactions formal and require a release of information to be signed. I also make sure the families are aware I am interacting with the other professional. I think transparency is important in these exchanges. I regularly must reinforce boundaries with other professionals, not all professionals have the same legal and ethical guidelines that we are required to follow as licensed mental health providers.

Heidi Gerard Kaduson, PhD, RPT-S

Limits must be set for safety or as needed. Setting limits with humor allows there to be continued respect and trust among the therapist, parents, and the child. A playroom is for the child. It is safe and it is where they can say anything, do anything, and feel anything without judgment. Therefore, when the door closes, the walls are the physical boundaries for their safety and my acceptance of the client exactly where they are – and joining the child with whatever they need – this allows the boundaries to be symbolically set as well. With parents, I give information as needed, but most importantly, I work with them each session for ten minutes alone to teach a specific parent training lesson that is to slowly shift their parenting methods to fit and enhance the parent/child interactions.

I have a rule that no parents are allowed in the playroom, and if a child wants to tell a parent something during the parent's initial ten-minute meeting, they must knock on the door and wait for someone to open it. I show the same respect to a child client when I reenter the playroom by knocking on the door first. But when a limit must be set to clearly define a boundary (i.e., all toys stay in the playroom), I will joke about it so that the child doesn't feel like they asked or did something wrong. The need for a child to take something home is covering another need that I must explore with them. There is only one strong limit that I set, and that is when I hand over the Nerf dart guns to shoot at a target. As I hand them the guns, I would say, "You can only shoot at the target in this room and not at yourself or me because we must all be safe". I am ready for the impulsive child to try to see what happens if they go to shoot at anything other than the target. I grab the guns, put them in the bucket, and then quickly place the bucket of guns outside the door, and replace them with something else to throw. The next week, the child can use the guns as instructed. In my entire career, no child has ever shot at himself or me after the limit setting is provided. Boundaries and limits are important and make children feel safe.

Jennifer Lefebre, Psy.D., RPT-S

During the intake, I explain to families that the play therapy rooms are special and for therapy sessions only, and that there are toys and art supplies available in the waiting room while waiting for their therapist or for siblings to enjoy while waiting. The only directives or boundaries I have within the play therapy room are that we are gentle with each other and gentle with the toys. At times these boundaries are broken, and a child will take a toy home, or I will find one in the waiting area. Usually the parents are great about reinforcing this boundary. I will remind my client how important the toys are – usually each client has a favorite that they use. I will ask what it would be like if that toy wasn't in the playroom, and we can talk briefly about it.

The most difficulty boundary for me to enforce regards the use of cellphones. I have had parents and caseworkers checking their phones frequently during family or conjoint sessions, even after discussing this with them. This is a catch-22, as I understand that some have additional children not in the session, or a family member that is ill, and I understand that emergency situations are different. I typically have to remind adults more than children, to keep their phone use limited during family sessions. I believe this violates the safety and security of the child in therapy sessions, particularly because I am doing trauma and attachment work, and it breaks my heart to see a child look up at their parent in session to meet their cellphone instead of their eyes.

Clair Mellenthin, MSW, RPT-S

I feel that having clear expectations with regards to boundaries are important in the clinical field – as this helps to prevent burnout, manipulation, and triangulation. In my office, we have very clear guidelines and office policies that outline payment, session time and availability, 24-hour cancellation, and charges for no-show appointments that new and prospective clients are told from the beginning. Our office manager also requests a valid credit card before scheduling a new appointment and the client is told the card will be charged in full if they miss the appointment. In my initial parent consultation, we discuss confidentiality, what this looks like when working with a minor, as well as the difference between confidentiality and secret-keeping between parents. I set clear expectations for their involvement in their child's therapy as well as have them sign a release of information to be able to talk freely with other members of the treatment team, such as a pediatrician, psychologist, psychiatrist, and teacher,. We also discuss appropriate means of communication and the reasons why I do not give out my personal cell phone number or engage on social media with past or present clients.

In the playroom, setting clear limits, boundaries, and expectations is also important. In my very first session with a child, before doing anything else or engaging in an activity, we will discuss confidentiality and the limits of confidentiality in clear, child-based language to be sure that the child client understands what this means, and how it may affect them. This is a critical component of child psychotherapy that I feel at times is neglected or misunderstood. It is not enough to describe this to the adult parent or caretaker. Our child clients deserve the respect and time it takes to help them understand this. Too often, in various family and play therapy trainings I have facilitated, I have had therapists ask why this is necessary, or report feeling worried if they talk about this with a child, it may discourage them from disclosing abuse or neglect. This is a serious ethical and clinical issue that, as supervisors, we need to be sure we are training our supervisees and clinicians in our field about.

When I set boundaries with a child client, I try to be clear, firm, kind, and nurturing. As an adult, there is already a power differential in place and my job is to always model a secure attachment style in my interactions with children and their parents. Sometimes setting a boundary is helping a child regulate before doing anything else, as they are dysregulated and destructive. Other times, this occurs when I send a very clear verbal message saying, "Stop" and following the ACT limit setting strategy (Landreth, 2002). Yet, at other times, this can be diffused using playfulness and humor, sprinkled with validation and acceptance, which I find can be one of the best ways at setting boundaries with my child clients.

Akiko J. Ohnogi, PsyD

I believe maintaining boundaries is extremely important, not only for the clients but also for the play therapist. It is a topic that I incorporate in classes and workshops and I often hear of countless reports of failure in treating the client properly or burnout of the clinician due to the play therapist's inability to maintain appropriate boundaries with clients, parents, and/or other professionals. The following is a list of some of the limits I consider worthwhile or necessary within the therapeutic working relationship.

1 I clearly inform my clientele and other professionals of my office hours and only respond to inquiries and requests during those hours.
2 I clarify my professional role and specify what I can and cannot do and to what extent I can be of support.
3 Everything that I explain to clients, parents, and other professionals is relayed using both verbal and nonverbal communication (information in writing) that communicates acknowledgement and understanding of the other's request.
4 I am always friendly and maintain a professional manner. I do not become personally involved with clients outside of the sessions, and I do not divulge personal information, even when asked.
5 I do not give clients gifts or cards; however, I am fine with clients sending them to me. Likewise, I accept small seasonal gifts from children that are handmade. I will not give anything in return other than saying "Thank you".
6 I do not attend any private activities that I am invited to (e.g., child's school concert, birthday party, graduation). I instead use the opportunity therapeutically to work on issues such as their need for approval, feelings of rejection, and lack of self-worth.
7 I do not extend the session time even if there is no one scheduled after the current client.
8 I am consistent in implementing limit setting during sessions if there are boundary issues, whether it be with the child or parent.
9 I conduct parent consultations only during parent consultation time and not during the child's session time.
10 I do not conduct therapy with parents as part of the child's treatment. Consultation sessions with parents is just that, a consultation, and not therapy for the parents as individuals.

Mary Anne Peabody, EdD, RPT-S

Small communities and rural social work are unique practice arenas. I am actually a very private person rarely mixing anything in my personal life with my professional life. In fact, if you have met anyone in my family, you are part of a very rare circle of people. Even in today's social media world, my sharing and responding is carefully crafted and infrequent.

I realize this behavior is greatly influenced by practicing for many years in a small community where only a few child therapists existed. At the time, I was the only registered play therapist supervisor and simultaneously my husband and I were raising my own two children. Like most therapists, my disclosure statement did address issues of maintaining boundaries around seeing each other in the community, gift giving, or invitations to social events. I communicated to parents only over the phone or in person not by email or text messaging.

The "goldfish effect" (Riebschleger, 2007) was part of our lives, meaning I had to constantly manage intersecting roles where both my professional and personal actions were observed and where it seemed that everyone was connected in one way or another. While most unanticipated encounters with clients and families were innocuous and did not pose a problem, I spent a lot time setting appropriate boundaries to protect my clients' interests to the greatest extent possible. Even so, despite setting and maintaining consistent boundaries, there were a handful of experiences over the years where my professional and personal worlds did collide. While I managed these incidents, I think living in the same small community you practice in, should if possible, be avoided.

Setting boundaries with clients in the playroom seems the easiest part of this question, as I have very clear and theoretical sound reasons for how I handle limit setting or touch. If I can be clear and consistent it contributes to needed safety. This constancy and consistency is therapeutically part of my theoretical training, embedded in my treatment approaches, and thereby contributes to treatment success.

Dee Ray, PhD, RPT-S

An essential construct within child-centered play therapy is the belief and practice of returning responsibility (Landreth, 2012; Ray, 2011). The belief behind returning responsibility is that all persons are capable and hold the ability to move toward self- and other-enhancing behaviors. In the playroom, I practice returning responsibility to children through facilitating decision-making and encouraging a positive self-concept. Therapeutic responses such as, "in here you can decide", "that's up to you", or "you figured that out on your own" set the stage for children to learn just what they are capable of doing. When children cross boundaries or engage in behaviors that are designed to elicit the therapist exerting control over the child, I believe that limit-setting is the most effective response to maintaining boundaries.

In the ACT technique (Landreth, 2012) of limit-setting, I am able to empathically respond to the child through acknowledging their feelings or needs ("you love being here with me ...") while I am communicating the boundary ("but I am not for kissing") and targeting an alternative ("you can give me a hug"). This limit-setting technique is helpful to me because I often feel torn in wanting to give the child what the child seems to really want, especially when it is a loving intention. With ACT, I am able to still journey with the child by connecting with the person of the child in recognition of feelings, thoughts, desires, and intentions. Even though I need to set a limit, I am still able to relationally connect with the child. ACT returns responsibility to the child because I state the limit and then it is the child's decision regarding how to respond to the limit.

I use ACT in all boundary situations for both children and adults. I find it to be effective across the life span, and again it helps me maintain my need for relationship with clients and systemic partners while honoring the need for boundaries between us. With parents, I might use ACT in examples such a when they are demanding my time beyond reason or when they impose on their child's play therapy time in responses such as "You are really struggling and needing support right now, but I am unavailable to talk each evening, we can schedule a time once per week between sessions", or "You are hurting for your family and your child, but the time right now is for your child, we can schedule a time for us later in the week". When ACT does not seem to work to help parents maintain boundaries, I engage in caring confrontation with parents in order to ascertain how to meet their needs while keeping appropriate boundaries.

Jessica Stone, PhD, RPT-S

A critical part of therapeutic work is the initial meetings. The intake is a place to not only gather information and complete the necessary forms but also begin the process of the family being oriented to your practice. This is the time and place for many things to be explained and "front-loaded". This process sounds simple, but at times, it is quite complicated initially as the clinician has a lot to determine early in their practice. Front-loading information allows the family to make informed decisions about the services the clinician provides, allows for questions to be asked and addressed, and sets the structure for important boundaries to be communicated.

The play therapist has a lot of important aspects to determine for him/herself. How long will sessions last? How will the caregivers and/or other family members be involved (when, how often, why, etc.)? Beyond the legal requirements of HIPAA and confidentiality, how will information be shared or not shared and with whom? How will play therapy be explained and what can be discussed in advance to avoid the inevitable questions later such as "I paid how much for you to play basketball with my child?".

Once a practitioner understands the state and ethical requirements within their discipline, the rest should be carefully explored and defined by the individual clinician. Even when there are agency parameters, ultimately the clinician is responsible for the care provided and conversations may need to be held to ensure the quality of care is paramount. I liken it to playing a game. If all the players understand the same set of rules, the game tends to go relatively smoothly. If players are understanding different rules and have differing expectations of the course of play, then a whole host of emotional and behavioral reactions can follow. The more the clinician can clearly communicate the boundaries, expectations, and services provided at the onset of treatment, and then remain consistent with what was communicated, the more positive the process will be for all involved.

Daniel Sweeney, PhD, RPT-S

In terms of setting boundaries with children in the playroom, it is a simple awareness and practice of therapeutic limits. I would refer to a previous publication, Sweeney and Landreth (2009), and suggest several rationales for setting limits, which include the following:

- Limits define the boundaries of the therapeutic relationship.
- Limits provide security and safety for the child, both physically and emotionally.
- Limits demonstrate the therapist's intent to provide safety for the child.
- Limits allow the therapist to maintain a positive and accepting attitude toward the child.
- Limits allow the child to express negative feelings without causing harm, and the subsequent fear of retaliation.
- Limits promote and enhance the child's sense of self-responsibility and self-control.
- Limits provide for the maintenance of legal, ethical, and professional standards. (pp. 132–133)

I use Landreth's (2012) A-C-T limit-setting model in the playroom, which includes three steps: (1) **a**cknowledge the child's feelings, wishes, and wants; (2) **c**ommunicate the limits; and (3) **t**arget acceptable alternatives. An example involving a child wanting to paint my arm in the playroom would sound like, "I know it seems like fun to paint my arm, but my arm is not for painting, the paper is for painting".

With parents, setting boundaries with them is fundamentally the same as with non–play therapy clients. However, there are two issues that come to mind in the context of play therapy. The first is that I need to educate parents about confidentiality and privilege. There are, of course, the normal limits to confidentiality (abuse, intended harm, etc.). With child therapy, I want to fully acknowledge the parent's right to privilege (a legal concept) but also stress that the child should have a level of confidentiality. Like any client, children will be reticent to disclose if they think that I will discuss every detail with parents. I tell parents that they can ask me any question at all and that I will tell them all details around issues of safety – however, I prefer that the give honor to their child's (nonlegal) right to confidentiality.

With caseworkers, I want to honor their role in cases, recognizing the legal and ethical rights of all involved parties. It is clear that I will need written and signed authorization to speak with any related party to a child case.

It is the play therapist's responsibility to be aware of legal and ethical issues, which can vary from state to state (Sweeney, 2015). This applies directly to issues of boundaries. Play therapists are encouraged to be familiar with the APT's (2019) *Play Therapy Best Practices*.

References

Association for Play Therapy (2019). *Play therapy best practices: Clinical, professional & ethical issues.* https://www.a4pt.org/resource/resmgr/publications/best_practices_-_ sept_2019.pdf.

Grant, R. J. (2017). *AutPlay therapy for children and adolescents on the autism spectrum: A behavioral play-based approach.* Routledge.

Kolmes, K. (2012). Social media: What's your policy? *Good Practice: Tools and Information for Professional Psychologists,* Spring/Summer, 10–18.

Kolmes, K., & Taube (2016). Client discovery of psychotherapist personal information online. *Professional Psychology: Research and Practice, 47,* 147–154.

Kottman, T., & Meany-Walen, K. (2016). *Partners in play: An Adlerian approach to play therapy.* American Counseling Association.

Landreth, G. L. (1991). *Play therapy: The art of the relationship.* Accelerated Development Inc. Publishers.

Landreth, G. L. (2002). *Play therapy: The art of the relationship* (2nd ed.). Brunner-Routledge.

Landreth, G. L. (2012). *Play therapy: The art of the relationship* (3rd ed.). Routledge.

Ray, D. (2011). *Advanced play therapy: Essential conditions, knowledge, and skills for child practice.* Routledge.

Riebschleger, J. (2007). Social workers' suggestions for effective rural practice. *Families in society: The journal of contemporary human services,* 88(2), 203–213.

Sweeney, D. (2015). Play therapy and the legal system. In K. O'Connor, C. Schaefer, & L. Braverman (eds.), *Handbook of play therapy* (Vol. 2). Guilford Publications.

Sweeney, D., & Landreth, G. (2009). Child-centered play therapy. In K. O'Connor & L. Braverman (Eds.), *Play therapy theory and practice: Comparing theories and techniques* (2nd ed., pp. 123–162). Wiley.

VanFleet, R. (2014). *Filial therapy: Strengthening parent-child relationships through play* (3rd ed.). Professional Resource Press.

18 How Do You Prevent Burnout and Compassion Fatigue?

Jeff Ashby, PhD, RPT-S

When I consider burnout and compassion fatigue, I am reminded of the broader construct of emotional competence. In my play therapy work, I am not so much trying to prevent burnout and compassion fatigue as I am trying to maintain emotional competence. Koocher and Keith-Spiegel (2008) define emotional competence as the,

> therapists' ability to emotionally contain and tolerate the clinical material that emerges in treatment, their willingness and skill at detecting the intrusion of personal biases into their work, and their capacity for self-care in the context of the difficult work of psychotherapy.
>
> (p. 71)

One of the primary ways I use to bolster my ability to "tolerate the clinical material that emerges in therapy" (and avoid compassion fatigue) is consultation. I have inspiring colleagues with whom I consult regularly. They are encouraging, they know me well, they are all amazing play therapists, and they help me synthesize clinical material into a clearer conceptualization of the client and a more effective treatment plan. These same amazing colleagues help me guard against the intrusion of my own issues and biases into my work. They are honest, supportive, and firm. I'm deeply grateful for this community and, if you don't have them, I urge you to work to find similar colleagues!

Koocher and Keith-Spiegel (2008) specifically mention the importance of self-care. Self-care can take numerous forms. Often self-care involves social components. For me, this is being with family and friends, near and far. Self-care can also include avocations and pursuits that are life-giving. I love to exercise, to be outside, to play music, to travel, and to share these things with the people I love. Finally, self-care is often enhanced by meaning making, returning to the things that are most important. I have a community of people who share my Christian faith with whom I can lock arms in every season of life. When I begin to move toward a place of disillusionment, I'm buoyed by reminders from Adlerian psychology that "people are creative, resourceful, and whole" (Kottman, personal communication, November 25, 2019) and from Martin Luther King Jr. (1968) that "The arc of the moral universe is long but it bends toward justice".

Robert Jason Grant, EdD, RPT-S

I began my professional work career as a hotline investigator for children's services working in a rural county in Missouri. This was my first professional job after I completed my bachelor's degree in psychology. I learned quickly that I needed to disengage from work and not take it home or I was going to become an unhealthy person. This experience equipped me well for understanding and implementing self-care and how to leave my work at the office which helped me when I began private practice. I worked in this position for one year and I was forced to critically examine compassion fatigue and burnout due to the high and consistent levels of negative human situations I was working with. I would conceptualize preventing burnout and addressing compassion fatigue as part of self-care. The larger picture of taking care of yourself as a lifestyle, protects against many unhealthy pitfalls including but not limited to burnout and compassion fatigue.

Skovholt and Trotter-Mathison (2016) stated that self-care means finding ways to replenish the self. The result is more important than the method. A major goal for professional self-care is to develop attitudes and activities that serve as natural endorphin boosters and stress hormone reducers. Self-care should focus in part on producing feelings of zest, peace, euphoria, excitement, happiness, and pleasure. Beginning private practice work I had a good awareness and process of self-care in my life and I have continued to refine the process. Some of the self-care strategies I have incorporated include making sure I schedule a full-hour lunch break in my day, and I don't participate in office work during the lunch break. I start my workday with a favorite drink. I have created self-care sand trays at work when I have had a particularly rough day, I might create a sand tray to express stress or negative emotions. I have a bowl of sensory and fidget toys at my desk that are just for me to use as needed.

I have also found that it helps to have other therapists to vent frustrations with. This has been an informal part of every clinic I have worked in and I have found this to be beneficial for other therapists as well as myself. Some therapists I know attend their own therapy for the purposes of self-care. Additionally, I make sure to get physical activity into my week and make time for uninterrupted downtime. I regularly implement activities such as prayer time and mediation, and try to pay attention to my work/home life balance. Self-care is an individualized lifestyle approach, with special attention to making sure it's maintained, consistent, and not optional.

Heidi Gerard Kaduson, PhD, RPT-S

There are many ways to prevent burnout, and self-care is the first priority. I have the ability to work long hours, but I always include at least two hours a day for exercise or play with my grandsons. Dancing in the morning is not only fun but invigorating. As I have been a play therapist for many years, and in my own therapy, I have always been focused on whether something I am doing is good for me. I don't take cases home in my head, and I have realistic expecta-tions about how much help I can be. My own trauma history has helped me understand and to be aware of possible triggers as I treat children and thus boundaries are set. Having a life that you love, as well as a passion for your work, allows for you to avoid burnout and/or compassion fatigue. Everyone has their own limits, and everyone should be in therapy themselves – understanding the importance of both of these prevent burnout from happening.

In addition, I don't take every case that comes in for referral. If there are problems in the intake, then I will not meet the child. I make sure I cover most of the issues and most of the historical aspects of the child I am about to see. If there is ongoing conflict, or the parents are demanding to be informed how long this therapy will take, I generally tell them that I never know because it is a process. If they don't like my response, I refer them elsewhere. Giving yourself permission to say no to certain clients can prevent future stress and help avoid compassion fatigue and burnout.

Jennifer Lefebre, PsyD, RPT-S

It is a priority of mine to connect with my loved ones, which is a huge factor in preventing burnout. My husband Derek is my rock – we balance each other in every way. He encourages me to do my best and is my sounding board and big-gest fan. We try to have date nights when possible and add time for ourselves when we travel together for conferences. Spending time with him, even just knowing he's next to me or there for me, is vital to my self-care.

I also have special rituals with my children which are a vital part of my self-care. My daughter Brighton (22) and I go out for coffee on Mondays and Tacos on Tuesdays, and monthly mani-pedis. I have an ongoing Yahtzee tournament with my son Seamus (18), and we have started going to the gym together and running together weekly. My son Declan (11) and I bake together weekly; he wants to be a pastry chef. My bonus daughter Taylor (24) and I share recipes and funny memes and jokes, and my bonus son Dominic (22) and I have had some awesome math parties and great talks. Lastly, my bonus son Drake (7) and I love building LEGO bricks and doing science experiments together. We play board games or watch movies often as a family and take time for outdoor play such as disc golf or hiking. I made it a point to attend and volunteer at as many sports games as I could, as well as school concerts, and I volunteer for field trips or classroom whenever I can.

Music is one of my favorite things for my own self-care. I am a rock-star in my jeep, singing my heart out to anything from Lita Ford to Janis Joplin, or the Violent Femmes to AC/DC. I listen to music based on my mood and what I need to accomplish for the day, and I have several playlists that I use specif-ically in this regard – my favorite is my "On my way to testify" playlist. Music keeps my grounded and focused.

Physical health and well-being is vital for me in preventing burnout. I com-pete in obstacle course races (i.e., Spartan, Savage, Tough Mudder) as part of my self-care. Even after I was seriously injured (not in a race), I was motivated to work out and return to these races (not my only motivation to heal, of course). Additionally, I have met new people from all over the world and heard fascinating stories from others during these races. The support and encouragement from people during these races is amazing, everyone cheers each other on and assists one another when needed. Pushing myself to be stronger physically and mentally is important to my self-care.

Clair Mellenthin, MSW, RPT-S

Boundaries, boundaries, and more boundaries! This is a lesson I have had to learn over and over again throughout my 20-year career experience. I have had to learn that I am OK to love myself enough and to put my family first over my client's needs and desires. This may sound like a no brainer, but I think it's easy to let go of your boundaries in this field since we are here because we care deeply and passionately about helping others, especially vulnerable children. It's easy to want to work every night to fit all the kids on your caseload into your schedule or to never give yourself a day off because you have too many clients to schedule. I have learned that in each season of my life, there is a balancing act that I need to figure out how to keep me, my home, and my work stable. For example, when I was younger and had babies and young children at home, I made the decision to change to part-time work because I found that I needed those moments with my little ones just as much as they needed me. I was also very lucky to have a partner and husband who was totally supportive of this and could help fill in the gaps financially due to this change.

As the years have flown by, my schedule has changed several times as I try to find the right balance between home and work. I have also realized how critical it is to engage in self-care. Yes, getting a monthly pedicure is fabulous and one thing I do for myself, but it is the smaller moments of self-care that I have found are the most helpful. Giving myself permission to decompress after a long day before heading home to be Mom, lying in bed and reading the daily news while drinking a cup of tea or coffee a few minutes after my kids go to school in the morning, making date nights and time with my husband a huge priority, eating healthy foods, exercising, and seeking out my own therapy when I have needed it have been a few of the things I have found I need to keep motivated and present in my play therapy practice.

I have found for me, one thing that has helped to decrease compassion fatigue is to have a varied caseload of presenting problems, ages, and stages of clientele. I now work with a mixture of adult, teen, and child clients, and it varies from individual to family to group work. This has done wonders for my soul and brain, and helped me to be engaged, focused, and excited for the work I do. I also rely on and seek out supervision and consultation from mentors in the field and have a strong network of dear friends who also are play therapists whom I can count on to help me work through different challenges and experiences. I am so grateful to work in a practice where I can knock on the door of any of my colleagues and receive sound advice, a shoulder to cry on, and someone to help me process through these experiences.

Akiko J. Ohnogi, PsyD

This is a topic that is extremely important to me, as the play therapy association that I cofounded (Japan Association for Play Therapy) has been doing a lot of natural disaster trauma survivor support work since the 2011 Tohoku earthquake, tsunami, and nuclear reactor disaster. I believe it's extremely important to have strategies to prevent burnout and compassion fatigue when doing survivor support work. This became very clear to me following the experience I had when I was a member of a team of play therapists that the Association for Play Therapy sent to Sri Lanka to support children who were orphaned by the 2004 Indian Ocean earthquake and tsunami. It was a result of this experience that I developed and implemented strict guidelines regarding self-care to avoid the hazards of burnout when working in a caring profession.

A summary of the protocols I developed to prevent burnout and compassion fatigue for the survivor support interventionists include (1) work with and train under a group of professionals who are qualified for the support intervention and have an incident command structure for interventions and self-care; (2) work in pairs, utilizing the buddy system to support and asses each other's psychological and physical health, and remind each other to take breaks; (3) check-in with others before, during, and after going to a disaster area to assess psychological and physical fitness, and for any practical, or emotional support that might be needed; (4) incorporate daily self-care, attend mandatory vicarious traumatization prevention workshops utilizing play activities, and take time off from any disaster support work every six to eight weeks for at least one week at a time (Ohnogi, 2017).

One example that I use when explaining the importance of self-care is the typical announcement that is made on airplanes. When on a flight, one of the messages that all passengers receive is to place your own breathing apparatus on before helping anyone else, including your child. This is to ensure that you can breathe and be conscious to help others. If you neglect to ensure your own safety first, the danger of you losing consciousness prior to helping your child increases, placing both you and your child at risk. The same idea applies to those in a helping profession. If you are not doing well emotionally and physically, not only will the chances of you being able to help others decrease, but you may be placing yourself in danger of burnout.

Regardless of whether I am doing trauma survivor support work or not, I make sure that I implement many different types of self-care within my daily life. I would increase the amount of self-care whenever I feel I have had a taxing session or seen a difficult client. I consult with others for emotional and practical support, especially if I think my countertransference is being triggered. I also take frequent breaks and try to have multiple vacations scheduled throughout the year.

Mary Anne Peabody, EdD, RPT-S

After more than 35 years in the field, I am very aware of how I handle stress. I experience compassion fatigue in my body, my language, and in my interactions with others. When I become cynical or quick to react in unconventional ways or experience tenseness in my shoulders and neck, I know it is time to step back and reflect on what is occurring. In trying to make the world a better place, a toll is taken. It is true that years of hearing and holding trauma stories or being involved with vulnerable children and families has made me different than others (van Dernoot Lipskys & Burk, 2009).

However, the mere fact that I am still practicing after 35 years shows I have learned a few strategies to prevent burnout and compassion fatigue. Professionally I intentionally diversify tasks so that I have a mix of consultation, teaching, training, and writing, providing supervision, and being in supervision. As I look back over my career, there is a defined pattern whereby every eight to ten years I have either switched agencies or returned to higher education for another degree. Now as a full-time professor, I am subject to higher education organizational issues that can easily deplete my energy as I juggle teaching, service, and research in the underresourced public University system. Pragmatically, I am off contract in the summer and can choose whether I want to teach during that semester. More often than not, I choose not to teach during the summer semester so that I can have time to write and reflect, travel, participate in study groups, and spend as much time as possible playing outside during these precious few weeks.

I am someone who engages in gratitude reflections several times a day. I start and end every day with a few private minutes of reflection. I also participate three to four times a week in either a Pilates or strength training group class with a personal trainer. Thanks to Pilates, I have learned to breathe correctly and have found myself utilizing breathing several times a day. I am very serious about my sleep and make getting at least eight to nine hours of sleep a night a very high priority. It is quite rare to see me awake after 10 pm during the work week.

Finally, I am so very fortunate to be a grandmother of a delightful little boy who lives only 20 minutes away. This allows me pure playtime almost whenever I want it and being a grandparent is a remarkable experience. I loved every single moment of being a parent, even the difficult moments, and being a grandparent is an extension of my human capacity to love and give selflessly. I think it is so important for child therapists to spend time with children who are not our clients. Children are our best teachers about anything that truly matters.

Dee Ray, PhD, RPT-S

I have been a play therapist for almost 25 years, and I cannot say that I have always been successful at preventing burnout. The powerless state of children weighs daily on me. Working with children who are at the mercy of parents with significant problems, schools with damaging practices, and organizational systems that lack the will or knowledge to serve the best interests of children elicits feelings of sadness, hopelessness, and overresponsibility. There have been times in my career where I was burned out. For me, burnout occurs every few years when I have repeatedly chosen to put clients in the forefront of my awareness at work and at home, at the expense of taking care of my personal relationships. My signs of burnout include resentment toward my clients, friends, and family who need me or sometimes just want to connect with me to maintain our relationship. I know that when a friend asks to have lunch and my internal thought is "what do they need from me?" that I am in a burnout phase that has crept up on me. When I become aware of being in burnout, I typically take action to decrease my scheduled responsibilities and take time off for me. I spend time alone to recharge (the primary indicator that I am an introvert!), purposefully scheduling hours to be by myself with no responsibilities to others. I, then, intentionally schedule one-on-one time with friends and family to restart work-life balance. In burnout phases, I have found that I have to make deliberate attempts to schedule personal relationship time because I am not open to spontaneous interactions due to lack of energy and hyper-focus on professional responsibilities.

For most of my career, I have engaged in practices that prevent burnout and work successfully for me personally. I believe each play therapist has to find their way to what works best for their personal health. My primary practice to prevent burnout and compassion fatigue is to diversify my responsibilities. I am unable to only see clients in play therapy sessions and maintain an optimistic and balanced perspective. In addition to seeing clients, I teach, supervise, research, and engage in other types of mental health services such as assessment and process group work. On any given day, I perform multiple roles that allow me to fluidly move between cases in which things seem hopeless and lighter, less intensive tasks, resulting in greater balance for my professional optimism. I also attend to the gravity of my caseload. If I have seen a heavy load of clients who have disturbing backgrounds and circumstances, I will seek to take a client who is referred for moderate anxiety or a client whose parents just want to make sure their child is supported through an event such as divorce or recent surgery. This strategy helps me to be mindful that many children are growing up with typical developmental events and supportive systems.

Finally, I engage in self-care practices that are discussed in the literature and that I find to be personally helpful. Although it is a common suggestion, I believe that regular exercise is critical to maintaining good boundaries of self-care, an optimistic perspective, and physical health necessary for keeping up with children. I attempt to be mindful of what I am eating and how my desire to eat may be linked to my stress level. I seek out consultation with colleagues on cases that are hard for me. And I engage in hobbies that have absolutely nothing to do with working with children in order to give my mind a break from becoming overly concerned with the plight of clients and children in general.

Jessica Stone, PhD, RPT-S

Important beginnings to the prevention of burnout and compassion fatigue is self-knowledge, confidence, and healthy boundaries. If a therapist has a solid foundation which includes having explored one's own belief systems, goals, theoretical foundation, boundaries (personal and professional), and integrity, then it will become easier to portray each to others and seek environments which will nurture them. If a therapist has not explored these items, then the result is more muddied, the foundation is shaky, and the result is often unsatisfying for all involved.

Connecting with other professionals, whether informally in the community or formally through group supervision/consultation, can be very beneficial to prevent burnout and compassion fatigue. It can be incredibly helpful to decompress with someone who understands the work and is bound by confidentiality (it is important to include in your informed consent that you will seek professional consultation as needed). If the connection is more informal, be sure to have a conversation about the expectations of the consultation(s) with other professionals at the onset to ensure professionalism by all and to adhere to any and all discipline requirements of your state.

Another direction I have found to help with burnout is the involvement in new ventures. I am a person who wants to do and know more. I strive to better myself and positively impact my field. I want to learn and discover the obvious and the hidden aspects of many topics. Recently I set a challenge for myself to read collections from the founding theorists themselves. I have been writing and presenting quite a bit. In another area of growth, my husband and I created the Virtual Sandtray program for those people with whom and places in which a traditional sand tray process is not possible. It is amazing to work hard in a passion project which contributes to the field for the benefit of clients.

I also enjoy mentoring newer professionals. A previous boss frequently said that at a certain point in one's career it is important to "share one's cookies", meaning, pass on knowledge and experience to others. After almost three decades practicing in the mental health field it is exciting to have experience to share. For me, being involved in new ventures, learning, and sharing breathes new life into my work.

On a personal level, it is obvious to most that disconnecting from work, relaxing, vacationing, focusing on family, and working on pleasurable activities which are not work related are important. Time off should be taken for the good of the therapist and the positive impacts on their work. Frequently, parents are told to take care of themselves for the good of the family, the baby, and themselves. If they are depleted, they are less available in many ways to the people they are trying to prioritize. A play therapist's work is not very different either. If we do not build in time, remain cognizant of our own needs, maintain boundaries, and feel solid in our work's foundation, then the result will surely be burnout and compassion fatigue.

Daniel Sweeney, PhD, RPT-S

If play therapists have any expectation of an active and extended tenure, particularly if working with traumatized children, direct efforts for self-care must be a high priority. Compassion fatigue, a term popularized by Charles Figley (1995), is something that all play therapists are at risk for. Since my post-master's career started in the fields of forensic mental health and therapeutic foster care, I encountered many colleagues suffering from compassion fatigue and burnout. It has long been an awareness and concern of mine.

Additionally, during my doctoral program, the many self-inflicted stressors I encountered led to physical challenges that I contend with to the present day. Self-care is something that I passionately preach about to my own graduate students and supervisees.

For myself, preventing burnout is a matter of balance. I put a great deal of time and effort into my faith and my family. As an active Christian, I both give and receive spiritual support from my faith family. As a husband, father, and grandfather, I both give and receive love from a wonderful family. Faith and family are not simple expenditures of time but rather a way of *being*. Additionally, I have chosen to be a counselor educator on a full-time basis and a practicing psychotherapist on a part-time basis. My practice is balanced between individuals [children, adolescents, and adults], couples, and families – and is strictly limited to five to eight clients per week. When I add professional presentations and writing to this mix, life has great potential to become overloaded. I rely on my own discernment and consultation [personal and professional] to avoid becoming too busy and thus susceptible to burnout.

In addition to my efforts to maintain balance, I engage in multiple self-care activities. The most important are mentioned in the previous paragraph, which is my investment in my faith and family. Additionally, I am invested in several self-care practices, such as ensuring adequate sleep (a minimum of eight to nine hours/night), engagement in my own personal sand tray work and other creative arts activities, spending time in nature, reading nonprofessional literature, listening to music, balanced eating, moderate exercise, meditation, time with friends, humor, and personal therapy as needed.

Some play therapy–specific literature that I have enjoyed and recommend to my students and supervisees include Maschi (2015), Norcross and Drewes (2009), and Ryan and Cunningham (2007).

References

Figley, C. (Ed.). (1995). *Compassion fatigue: Coping with secondary traumatic stress disorder in those who treat the traumatized.* Brunner/Mazel.

King, M. L. (1968). Remaining awake through a great revolution. Speech given at the National Cathedral. https://kinginstitute.stanford.edu/king-papers/publications/knock-midnight-inspiration-great-sermons-reverend-martin-luther-king-jr-10.

Koocher, G. P., & Keith-Spiegel, P. (2008). *Ethics in psychology and the mental health professions: Standards and cases* (3rd ed.). Oxford University Press.

Maschi, T. (2015). Professional self-care and the prevention of secondary trauma among play therapists working with traumatized youth. In N. B. Webb (Ed.), *Play therapy with children and adolescents in crisis* (4th ed., pp. 395–416). The Guilford Press.

Norcross, J., & Drewes, A. (2009). Self-care for child therapists: Leaving it at the office. In A. Drewes (Ed.), *Blending play therapy with cognitive behavioral therapy: Evidence-based and other effective treatments and techniques* (pp. 473–493). John Wiley & Sons Inc.

Ohnogi, A. (2017). Play-based interventions for children traumatized by natural and human-made disasters. In A. A. Drewes & C. E. Schaefer (Eds.), *Childhood anxieties, fears, and phobias: Use of play-based interventions and techniques* (pp. 223–243). Guilford Publications.

Ryan, K., & Cunningham, M. (2007). Helping the helpers: Guidelines to prevent vicarious traumatization of play therapists working with traumatized children. In N. B. Webb (Ed.), *Play therapy with children in crisis: Individual, group, and family treatment* (3rd ed., pp. 443–460). The Guilford Press.

Skovholt, T. M., & Trotter-Mathison, M. (2016). *The resilient practitioner: Burnout and compassion fatigue prevention and self-care strategies for the helping professions.* Routledge.

van Dernoot Lipsky, L., & Burk, C. (2009). *Trauma stewardship: An everyday guide to caring for self while caring for others.* Berrett-Koehler Publishers.

19 How Do You Include Play in Your Play Therapy Supervision?

Jeff Ashby, PhD, RPT-S

The short answer to the question is that I use play in my play therapy supervision in lots of ways at lots of times. One consideration in the use of play in play therapy is the developmental level of the supervisee (from novice to advanced) and the stage of the supervision (Stoltenberg & Delworth, 1987). I generally approach supervision from Bernard's (1997) discrimination model. The discrimination model frames the supervisor as having three primary roles, teacher, counselor, and consultant – and three main foci in supervision, client conceptualization, intervention, and personalization. Bernard notes that this 3 × 3 matrix of supervision allows for any of the foci or supervision goals to be addressed in any of the supervision roles.

I use play therapy supervision activities at all stages of supervision. For instance, in the beginning phase of supervision I might use play therapy to facilitate the development of the supervisory relationship. I also use play therapy supervision with all levels of supervisees. With beginning play therapists, I may use play therapy in supervision to model techniques and reinforce the paradigm of play as the medium of change (Mullen et al., 2007). In similar fashion, I may use play therapy in each of the supervisory roles (teacher, counselor, and consultant) and to address each supervisory foci (conceptualization, intervention, and personalization). Play therapy activities in supervision are valuable for lots of reasons, not the least of which is they help develop playfulness. One of the things I love about the serious practice of play therapy is that it is fun! One of my goals in supervision is to keep that fun and using play therapy in play therapy supervision is one of the ways I strive to do that.

Because I regularly use play therapy in my supervision of play therapists, I include a description of these supervisory experiences in my informed consent for supervision (Thomas, 2007). As Mullen et al. (2007) note, some supervisees may be less comfortable with or feel vulnerable with the expressive processes inherent in many play therapy supervision activities. As a result, in my supervision informed consent I share the rationale for use of play therapy in supervision and outline the parameters of the supervisory relationship. I also need to be alert to the possibility of appropriate referral to personal counseling when using play therapy in supervision. Because play therapy activities and techniques (e.g., sand tray) can sometimes lead to personal insights at a deep level, the supervisees may be personally affected in ways they did not anticipate. Clarifying in informed consent, and being prepared in session, to facilitate appropriate referrals is extremely important.

Robert Jason Grant, EdD, RPT-S

If I were supervising someone who was not interested in or pursuing play therapy, I would likely not include much play in the supervision process. Currently, and for the past few years, all my supervision has involved practitioners who wanted to pursue becoming a Registered Play Therapist (RPT), thus the supervision time involved different aspects of play. Drewes and Mullen (2008) highlighted several ways to incorporate play and play interventions into the supervision process. I have often referred to their work for incorporating play into the supervision experience.

Involving play might include conducting play therapy supervision in a play therapy room and asking supervisees to participate in a play intervention connected to something we might be exploring in supervision. I recall working with a supervisee who was struggling with a child's behaviors. The child was very hyperactive, required many limits, and created a bit of chaos in play sessions. The supervisee was becoming stressed with the client's behaviors to the point of dreading when the child was coming in for a session. I had my supervisee complete a sand tray describing all the things he could think of about the client who was challenging him with their behavior. Then the supervisee completed a second sand tray describing all the things he could think of for why the client's behaviors bothered him. Finally, the supervisee completed a third tray describing all the things he could think of for reasons the client might be having these behaviors. This was a powerful processing intervention for my supervisee. It seemed to help him let go of looking at the child as a source of stress and helped him empathize with the child, especially when the child presented challenging behaviors.

I often reference Ray's (2011) four-step process of supervision as a guide when providing play therapy supervision: (1) skill-focused – focus on skill development while communicating empathy, unconditional positive regard, and genuineness; (2) experimentation and questioning – explore supervisees' thoughts about the philosophy of play therapy and congruence; (3) philosophical decision-making transformed into practice – supervisee adopts a philosophical approach to play therapy and supervision becomes more collaborative; and (4) person of play therapist emerges as professional – supervision becomes consultation, often initiated by the supervisee to explore the self in relationship to play therapy. I think play and play interventions have a place in any of the four processes. I try to give special consideration to where we are in the supervision process and what play intervention would be appropriate to enhance the supervisee's growth.

Heidi Gerard Kaduson, PhD, RPT-S

I believe in the therapeutic powers of play itself. I believe play therapy supervision must be playful and done with humor or techniques so that supervisees are comfortable and open to diversity and change without feeling the need to do it all correctly. Making mistakes has been the key to allowing children and supervisees to understand that perfectionism doesn't help to make a good play therapist; flexibility is the key. Bubble blowing, shaving cream, and other fun interventions that allow for mess and silly play begin most of the supervision sessions. By giving permission to play during supervision, we are encouraging the therapeutic powers of play to become ingrained in the supervisees. They learn more while having fun, and they appreciate this type of supervision because it is not focused on criticism but more focused on the supervisee gaining insight and understanding of themselves, play, and the power it has for children.

In supervision, we make up rating scales for how we think we did on certain sessions, and with humor we can play it out in supervision to see if the rating can become better or worse. Supervision in play therapy must be playful and techniques used so the therapist will understand how a child might feel under the same circumstances which we role play in supervision. In some supervision groups, I break up the group into dyads or groups of four, and they are required to work together and create a play therapy environment to help certain types of children. They must produce a process that they can role play or demonstrate and/or teach techniques that we will all experience while doing the supervision group. Learning, laughing, and creating proves to be very helpful to all of us.

Jennifer Lefebre, PsyD, RPT-S

I was blessed to have experienced play-based supervision during my doctoral training at Astor Home, where Athena Drewes was the training director at the time. The expressive arts became a natural part of supervision for me, and now as a supervisor I incorporate music, nature, play, and the expressive arts in supervision consistently. Teaching and training others inspires me, and I attempt to use creative approaches whenever possible.

I love holding supervision on the patio by the river outside of my office. Incorporating the sounds and sites of nature, as well as doing some gardening or finding stones, has been a great way to add self-care into supervision. We have seen bald eagles swooping for trout right in front of us, and once there was a deer by the river. Nature adds an element of grounding and openness that can't be found indoors.

Music is one of my favorite things in general, so, of course, it isn't any different in supervision. Finding a song that represents the clinical week has been a fun way to start supervision, or a song that reflects how you are transitioning out of the work week and into the weekend. Playing with musical instruments is fun in supervision too!

Creating a vision/self-care board on the back of a clip board has been something I have used in supervision. This has been a great way to get to know and experience my supervisees' professional goals and personal self-care, so that I can better support them in their growth as a play therapist.

And, of course, making time to play! My current supervisee Mr. Mike and I will play games like *Exploding Kittens* or *Throw, throw burrito* to have fun for a few minutes during supervision. This is so much fun and allows for a release and laughter, especially when tackling tough cases in supervision.

Clair Mellenthin, MSW, RPT-S

The play-based learning I use predominantly in supervision are sand tray and expressive arts. I supervise from a psychodynamic perspective and try to help my supervisees understand issues of countertransference and transference, their own parallel process of learning and healing occurring, as well as teaching new play therapy skills by learning and experiencing them firsthand. I supervise a wide variety of clinicians presently, from graduate interns at my agency practice, online play therapy supervision with new and seasoned licensed clinicians, to agency department heads trying to implement play therapy into their clinics and agencies. Depending on their clinical needs and experiences, the use of play will vary, but it is critical to put into supervision practice.

As with clients, the use of expressive arts and a sand tray can help facilitate new insight, awareness of self in the environment, and access to the unconscious – all of which are critical supervision issues that need to be addressed. I also find that the supervisee-supervisor relationship is enhanced when utilizing play as compared to merely talking about cases or clinical issues. It is through the direct experience that you can really access and understand the therapeutic powers of play. I also use play to role play and practice different models of play therapy, as the supervisee is learning new ways of engaging and treating their clients in psychotherapy.

Akiko J. Ohnogi, PsyD

The model of supervision I use with supervisees is an integration of the Discrimination Model and Lifespan Model (Bernard & Goodyear, 2018). I help supervisees continue to grow across their professional developmental lifespan by addressing their needs and supervision foci. I alternate my supervisory role as teacher, counselor, or consultant while prescribing play-based techniques and interventions that I assess as most useful for the individual at that time.

I also utilize trauma-informed supervision, being aware of the potential impact that a client's trauma has for the supervisee (Knight, 2018). The supervisee might be affected by vicarious traumatization from sessions with clients, as well as, the supervisee's own trauma being triggered by a client and/or supervision. I emphasize physical, psychological, and emotional safety for the supervisee and myself as the supervisor. I also help the supervisee experience a sense of control and empowerment. I believe that supervision needs to be relational (safe), relevant (developmentally matched), repetitive (patterned), rewarding (pleasurable), rhythmic (resonant with biology), and respectful (child, family, culture) (Perry, 2006).

I also believe that incorporation of play-based activities in play therapy supervision is extremely important and necessary. Experience and experiential activities can foster access to integration of holistic brain processes by engaging the supervisees senses, feelings, and thoughts; facilitate the supervisees self-awareness and self-reflections; and enhance their conceptualization of clients and insight into the child-play therapist relationship. My role as the supervisor would be to present the activity and be witness to the creation – making sure to observe nonverbal communication and process the creation with the supervisee.

Play-based activities may elicit experiences and feelings that are out of the supervisee's awareness. When utilizing play in supervision I try to consider the following:

1   The supervisee's emotional developmental level.
2   Selection of activities with intentionality based on the supervisee's need and level of processing.
3   Respecting the supervisee's choice to decide on their level of participation and sharing.

I also make sure that the supervisee is comfortable with what they use in an activity. As expressive mediums impact individuals differently based on the degree of control over the medium, each supervisee will experience this differently. I often use clay/Play-Doh, sand, miniatures, and drawing with supervisees, while having all toys and materials used in play therapy available for use in supervision.

Mary Anne Peabody, EdD, RPT-S

My theory of supervision is strongly influenced by the developmental model of Stoltenberg, McNeill, and Delworth (1998) and the discrimination model of Bernard and Goodyear (2018). I was fortunate to achieve a Certificate of Advanced Study in Play Therapy and Clinical Supervision under the direction of the late Dr. Marijane Fall, a play therapy researcher and gifted teacher. She modeled playful supervision for her students in a variety of ways and I am forever grateful for her guidance and mentorship. She and coauthor, Dr. John Sutton, also one of my professors, published the book *Clinical Supervision: A Handbook for Practitioners* (2004), which included a full segment on supervision and sand tray work.

A few years later when Athena Drewes and Jodi Mullen edited book, *Supervision Can be Playful* (2008) was published, I devoured every page with a voracious appetite. I even contemplated doing my dissertation on the topic of playful supervision and immersed myself in this area of literature for a while. Along the same time, I discovered LEGO® SERIOUS PLAY® (LSP) as a methodology used in business and higher education contexts and could readily see the connections and possibilities in clinical supervision. I began using an adapted version of the full LSP methodology in my teaching and clinical supervision practice as a way to socialize therapists into the play therapy field (Peabody, 2015). I strongly believe in active experiential learning for all age levels and take every opportunity to "learn though play" with my supervisees and adult students.

Whether it is through art, sand tray work or LSP, accessing the therapeutic powers of play in supervision is imperative (Schaefer & Drewes, 2014). I assert playful supervision should be required supervisory training content and considered a competency area of a well-trained play therapy supervisor.

Dee Ray, PhD, RPT-S

Play is a thread that is woven throughout my supervision approach in various ways. In a developmental supervision model (Ronnestad & Skovholt, 2013), early play therapist supervisees respond more effectively to a detailed, teaching role in which the supervisor offers education and concrete information to help guide the supervisee and reduce anxiety. During early supervision phases, I use role-play techniques to teach and practice skills. We discuss skills and then practice those skills through role-play in which sometimes I take the therapist role and sometimes I take the child role. Often, I will engage in role-play in the playroom to re-create play therapy session moments experienced by the supervisee. These role-plays can be a fun way to make supervision active and more realistic to the actual play therapy experience.

As supervisees become more experienced and are in need of deeper level processing of their role as a play therapist, I use expressive arts structured activities such as sand tray work, drawing, and arts/crafts materials. A few prompts for these activities include make a scene of you with this client, draw yourself as a play therapist, create the perfect play therapist, and create what a healthy work-life balance would look like for you. Expressive arts processing helps to bring out internal conflicts, struggles with self-regard, and relational challenges which are frequent issues of concern for play therapist supervisees. In addition to using planned play activities in supervision, I offer play materials/toys in my office for any spontaneous need for play that may arise. I have a small sand tray with a few nature items, fidget toys, magic wands, and multiple manipulatives. These items are openly displayed in my office for supervisees to pick up at any given time during supervision sessions. Supervisees will often use toys as an adjunct to their verbal processing, to soothe themselves, or to reduce their anxiety while working through issues in supervision.

Jessica Stone, Ph.D., RPT-S

Supervision is such a vital part of a play therapist's work. In some areas, such as the United Kingdom, supervision is a requirement for mental health providers throughout one's career. In the United States, supervision is typically a requirement for those in training, but not beyond. Supervision is an important way to ensure that the clinician is not operating in a vacuum. It allows for a fresh set of eyes and perspective regarding clinical care.

A great deal of playfulness is incorporated into the supervision I provide. Just as with clients, the experience of supervision will be more beneficial to the supervisee if they feel heard, seen, understood, and accepted. These are universal human needs. The role of the supervisor is the attend to many layers simultaneously, including the care of the clients <u>and</u> the abilities and needs of the supervisee. Laughter and connection will deepen the relationship within supervision so the focus can be the client care and the supervisee's needs, and not about uncomfortable, forced interactions.

Playfulness within supervision can include laughing, connecting, and having playful banter, etc. Supervision can also include direct play, either to assist the supervisee with gaining familiarity with different modalities, to demonstrate specific concepts, and/or work through anything that would benefit the client that the supervisee is experiencing. Sometimes there is a fine line between supervision and therapy for the supervisee since many personal issues can come up in supervision. It is important that the primary focus for the supervision is client care and if the need for the supervisee to have individual therapy apart from supervision arises, the supervisor should discuss this with the supervisee.

Frequently supervision with me includes the demonstration of a variety of drawing techniques, some craft creation, digital play, game play, and situation/diagnosis-specific projects. I think it is important that supervision include items which are, as stated above, included to either increase familiarity, demonstrate concepts, or assist the therapist so s/he can better assist the client. It is not craft time for the supervisee, it is inclusion with purpose. Face-to-face supervision with me can also include traditional sand tray, Virtual Sandtray, a variety of apps determined to be therapeutically beneficial, and virtual reality.

Daniel Sweeney, PhD, RPT-S

This question is very well worded. It assumes that play therapy methods are already included in the play therapy supervision – as it should. I would consider it inappropriate to avoid using play and expressive methods in the supervision process. There are many possible interventions – I would recommend the reader consult with Drewes and Mullen (2008). A suggestion for a solid introduction to using expressive arts in supervision is an article by Purswell and Stulmaker (2015).

I primarily use sand tray therapy (Homeyer & Sweeney, 2017) methods for the supervision of play therapy. I have found that sand tray therapy can be very effective to evaluate issues of transference and countertransference (Morrison & Homeyer (2008). Just as clients are able to access deep emotional issues through sand tray therapy, supervisees can access affective issues in the supervision process (Gibbs & Green, 2008).

Supervision using sand tray therapy methods can be used in both individual and group supervision. When proving group supervision, I will often follow a model proposed by Anekstein, Hoskins, Astramovich, Garner, and Terry (2014):

1   Introduce supervisees to the sand trays and the available tools.
2   Ask the supervisees to close their eyes for a brief relaxation exercise of concentrating on their breathing.
3   Give supervisees the Bernard's (1979) Discrimination Model-based directive to reflect on specific clients with whom they are working and then reflect on the three foci of supervision (intervention, conceptualization, and personalization) of Bernard's Discrimination Model. Encourage them to use one, two, or all three components. Have supervisees use the sand tray to illustrate how they have been working with their clients.
4   Process the sand trays of the supervisees in the following steps:

   a   observe while the supervisees are creating the sand trays;
   b   ask the supervisees to name the theme of the sand trays;
   c   ask the supervisees which foci (intervention, conceptualization, or personalization) are being illustrated;
   d   ask supervisees to discuss the sand tray worlds and process from general to specific;
   e   invite the supervisees to give voices to the figurines;
   f   ask supervisees which foci of supervision (intervention, conceptualization, or personalization) identified by Bernard's (1979) Discrimination Model they now see in their sand trays after discussing them; and
   g   invite the supervisees to make any changes and rename the themes of the sand trays.

5   Ask the supervisees for any additional feedback.
6   Give the supervisees the option to photograph the sand tray.
7   Document the session and clean up materials. (p. 127)

While using sand tray methods in play therapy supervision is my primary approach, I have also used other expressive methods, including painting, collage work, clay and Play-Doh work, and the creation of mandalas.

References

Anekstein, A., Hoskins, W., Astramovich, R., Garner, D., & Terry, J. (2014). Sandtray supervision: Integrating supervision models and sandtray therapy. *Journal of Creativity in Mental Health, 9*(1), 122–134.

Bernard, J. M. (1997). The discrimination model. In C. E. Watkins, Jr. (Ed.), *Handbook of psychotherapy supervision* (pp. 310–327). Wiley.

Bernard, J. M., & Goodyear, R. K. (2018). *Fundamentals of clinical supervision* (6th ed.). Pearson.

Drewes, A., & Mullen, J. (2008). *Supervision can be playful: Techniques for child and play therapist supervisors.* Rowman & Littlefield Publishers.

Fall, M., & Sutton, J. M. (2004). *Clinical supervision: A handbook for practitioners.* Pearson Publishing, Allyn and Bacon.

Gibbs, K., & Green, E. (2008). Sanding in supervision: A sand tray technique for clinical supervisors. In A. Drewes & J. Mullen (Eds.), *Supervision can be playful: Techniques for child and play therapist supervisors* (pp. 27–38). Rowman & Littlefield Publishers.

Homeyer, L., & Sweeney, D. (2017). *Sandtray therapy: A practical manual* (3rd ed.). Routledge.

Knight, C. (2018). *Trauma-informed supervision: Historical antecedents, current practice, and future directions.* The Clinical Supervisor. https://doi.org/10.1080/07325223.2017.1413607.

Morrison, M., & Homeyer, L. (2008). Supervision in the sand. In A. Drewes & J. Mullen (Eds.), *Supervision can be playful: Techniques for child and play therapist supervisors* (pp. 233–248). Rowman & Littlefield Publishers.

Mullen, J. A., Luke, M., & Drewes, A. A. (2007). Supervision can be playful, too: Play therapy techniques that enhance supervision. *International Journal of Play Therapy, 16,* 69–85.

Peabody, M. A. (2015). Building with purpose: Using LEGO® SERIOUS PLAY® in play therapy supervision. *International Journal of Play Therapy, 24*(1) 30–40.

Perry, B. D. (2006). Applying principles of neurodevelopment to clinical work with maltreated and traumatized children: The neurosequential model of therapeutics. In N. B. Webb (Ed.), *Working with traumatized youth in child welfare* (pp. 27–52). Guilford press.

Purswell, K., & Stulmaker, H. (2015). Expressive arts in supervision: Choosing developmentally appropriate interventions. *International Journal of Play Therapy, 24*(2), 103–117.

Ray, D. (2011). *Advanced play therapy: Essential conditions, knowledge, and skills for child practice.* Routledge.

Ronnestad, M., & Skovholt, T. (2013). *The developing practitioner: Growth and stagnation of therapists and counselors.* Routledge.

Schaefer, C. E., & Drewes, A. A. (2014). *The therapeutic powers of play: Twenty core agents of change* (2nd ed.). Wiley.

Stoltenberg, C. D., & Delworth, U. (1987) *Supervising counselors and therapists.* Jossey-Bass.

Stoltenberg, C. D., McNeill, B., & Delworth, U. (1998). *IDM supervision: An integrated developmental model for supervising counselors and therapists.* Jossey-Bass.

Thomas, J. T. (2007). Informed consent through contracting for supervision: Minimizing risks, enhancing benefits. *Professional Psychology: Research and Practice, 38,* 221–231.

20 How Do You Use Play Therapy Across the Life Span with Respect to Client Ages?

Jeff Ashby, PhD, RPT-S

I think play therapy is appropriate for clients across the life span. I have regularly used play therapy with adolescents. With adolescent (and older) clients my AdPT practice looks somewhat different from that of younger clients. While I still conceptualize the therapy as having four phases, the combination of directive and nondirective techniques are somewhat different. Because of adolescent, and older, clients' generally enhanced ability to verbalize their thoughts and emotions, nondirective interventions with my adolescent clients tends to be more verbal. However, I regularly use directive play therapy techniques with adolescents. Although sometimes initially reluctant, I've had great success using sand tray, expressive arts, kinesthetic movement, and other play techniques with adolescents. These techniques offer the same advantages for older clients as they do for younger children.

Especially in the last phase of play therapy, reorientation/reeducation, I often invite other family members into sessions. In these family sessions, I involve parents, caregivers, and/or siblings in the play interventions. I often design interventions to allow other members of the family a chance to try out interactional patterns or practice parenting skills. These family sessions, often including adult parents or caregivers, can give family members a chance to try out new behaviors and ways of relating to each other in a supportive and safe environment.

Finally, I love doing adventure therapy with clients of all ages, children, adolescents, and adults. Unlike traditional talk therapy, adventure therapy is "designed to kinesthetically engage clients on cognitive, affective, and behavioral levels" (Gass, Gillis, & Russell, 2012, p. 1). Using these play therapy techniques, often in groups, I can design adventure therapy interventions that have a metaphorical application to clients' lives.

Robert Jason Grant, EdD, RPT-S

Play therapy is a powerful tool across the life span. Play continues throughout the life span as an important construct because it fosters numerous adaptive behaviors including creativity, role rehearsal, and mind/body integration. Play is a holistic experience as it invites our total being into the process (Ward-Wimmer, 2003). There exists a fair amount of literature and trainings on using play therapy throughout the life span. Most play therapists understand that play therapy can be implemented with children through adults and is not exclusive to young children. I have often heard that the majority of play therapists work with children and the older a client becomes; the less play therapists work with them and less the client participates in a play therapy process. This would make logical sense as our culture seems to identify play as something that is only appropriate for young children. Although I work with clients throughout the life span, the majority of clients on my caseload have always been children – preschool through elementary age with preadolescents and adolescents being the next most common and adults making up the lowest percentage.

My work with adolescents is similar to my work with children when using play therapy. I might be child centered, integrative, or work out of a specific approach. I have used sand tray therapy, expressive play interventions, and various other play approaches with adolescents. In my work with adults I have implemented mostly play therapy techniques and interventions, I typically try to include play therapy with all my adult clients but some of them are too resistant or it does not seem like a good fit.

I recall a sand tray intervention I did with an adult male with cerebral palsy. He was struggling with depression mainly due to his disability and struggling to accept he had a disability. I introduced the sand tray and began with having him complete simple directive trays such as make a tray the describes you. He was hesitant to participate at first, but we had met several times and had developed good therapeutic relationship, so he was willing to try. After two completed sand trays he was very invested in the process. I have found this to be true of most adults when I get them to participate in a play therapy process. They will be hesitant at first but if they try, they typically like the results. The adult client with cerebral palsy completed several sand trays and was able to gain an acceptance of his disability and healthy view of himself which manifested in the progression of his sand tray work. Play therapy is certainly appropriate throughout the life span but may look differently depending on the age and developmental level of the client. If play therapists are willing to explore the possibilities, they will find another valuable tool in their toolkit for working with older children and adults.

Heidi Gerard Kaduson, PhD, RPT-S

I have treated children as young as 2 but only with respect to attachment disorder or severe separation anxiety. I don't believe there is a limit to how old a client can be to use play therapy. I have been training play therapists for about 25 years, and every workshop I do includes playful interventions and just playful moments. I noticed years ago that attendees would feel so good after the laughter that comes from many of these techniques. Teenagers are asked if they want to go in the playroom or office to "talk", and almost all chose the playroom. When given permission to play, many of these teenagers release much of their anger and resistance through throwing the *splatz* egg. Talking may happen during all the fun, but the process is self-healing for them. I truly believe that we all have within ourselves the ability to heal with the right environment and through play. If any person has experienced a trauma during childhood or even as an older person, I will ask them to first show me what happened by drawing, and then use release play therapy to slowly abreact the trauma until they have finished processing the event. If the play therapist is a true believer in the therapeutic powers of play, then the therapy will flow through play until the processing is complete.

Over the last 20 years, the view of play therapy as a treatment modality intended only for children has expanded to include adolescents (Schaefer, 2003), young adults (Kaduson, 2016), and geriatric populations (Fuss, 2010; Lindaman, 1994). Play remains an important part of many everyday experiences even when the mental age of a person is beyond the preoperational stage of development and can use language more abstractly (Piaget, 1936). Play is also a less direct avenue to the internal lives of children and adults (Erikson, 1993). It has been clinically shown that when play is presented, most people will join in or let go and allow the play to heal. Even with adults in rehabilitation centers, play therapy has been used to build trust among patients where there was none (Caldwell, 2003; Ward-Wimmer, 2003). Play therapy allows older children and adults to regress to an earlier developmental level if they need to work through something that happened during that stage of development. Play therapy can be used as a treatment for all ages, and the results are wonderful.

Jennifer Lefebre, PsyD, RPT-S

My first clinical job was at a halfway house where women served the last six to eighteen months of their sentences while receiving treatment for substance abuse, which was often the result of complex trauma in childhood through their adult years. I was 21, with a brand-new bachelor's degree in hand, and I decided these women needed to laugh and play. Our Sunday morning group therapy sessions were quickly dubbed the *Inner Child* groups. We would draw; play with clay; paint; play duck, duck, goose; write songs about recovery; dance; and do yoga. These women became more connected, more open, and started healing in a different way. The therapeutic powers of play were naturally there, within the walls of a historic jail built in 1812.

I remember fondly several women thanking me for not being afraid to be myself, for being authentic and real, and for playing with them. Several indicated that they didn't ever remember playing, as their childhoods had been chaotic and abusive. I knew nothing about play therapy in the year 2000, I did this because it felt right – and as I began my journey into graduate school, I quickly fell more in love with the power of play therapy.

Now, I use play therapy with not only the children, teens, and families I work with but with adult survivors of child abuse, first responders, and combat veterans. I have more tools and knowledge than I did back in 2000, but I still believe that being an authentic, real, playful therapist is truly the key to being an effective play therapist.

Clair Mellenthin, MSW, RPT-S

I use play therapy with all of my clients, regardless of age or presenting clinical issues. As I work with a wide variety of clientele, my play therapy language and interventions may change to meet the developmental needs of the age of my client. For example, with young children, calling the play therapy room and play therapy by its name is totally appropriate, however, when working with teens, I don't tend to use the same language about play therapy, even if we are doing the same thing. Most teens do not appreciate being thought of as younger or as a child, and I want to be sure my language reflects this. I may call the play therapy room the sand tray room or the arts and craft room, as developmentally, this is more appropriate to the age of the client. Play therapy is incredibly powerful when working with adolescent clients and their parents. Recent research (Green, 2010; Green et al., 2013) and publications such as Play Therapy with Preteens (Green et al., 2018) have focused on the impact of using play therapy with teens. I would strongly recommend familiarizing yourself with different theoretical perspectives and interventions to use with your tween and teen clients.

I utilize play therapy interventions consisting of expressive arts, movement, dance, sand tray, music, media, and technology with all clients at different therapeutic and life stages. I find these treatment approaches are incredibly powerful when working with adults, as doing so helps to decrease defense mechanisms, increase access to the unconscious, and improve mood and behavior (Garrett, 2014). Research has begun highlighting the positive impact that play therapy can have on adult psychotherapy from use in couples therapy and individual therapy. Kaduson (2016) recently published a chapter on using play therapy across the life span which is an invaluable resource in addition to Schaefer's (2003) book *Play Therapy with Adults*.

Akiko J. Ohnogi, PsyD

I use play therapy with all populations and ages from infancy to the elderly, including individual adults (Schaefer, 2003), adolescents (Schaefer & Gallo-Lopez, 2010), and children (Schaefer et al., 2008), as well as with couples, families, and in groups. The type of play therapy I use will vary with different ages. I always inform all my clients (regardless of their age) that play will be incorporated in their treatment – explaining why it is helpful and necessary before contracting with them to begin treatment. Basic information regarding the use of play therapy is outlined on my website and several other locations so that potential clients know in advance they will be asked to use play in their treatment.

Most people think of play therapy being used for children, but I have seen play therapy be useful for adolescents as they become more open when participating in an activity. They may be able to share more with drawing or using clay to express themselves. I have had many adolescents who initially refused to speak in sessions, but were happy to work on various play-based activities which not only helped in revealing their issues but also provided healing work.

Adults, especially those who have been traumatized, can benefit greatly from the use of play therapy in their psychological treatment, as the play activities will directly access the unconscious, nonverbal, sensory, and emotional memories of their trauma experience (Olson-Morrison, 2017). I have had many adult male clients working in the financial profession come to their sessions in their suit and tie initially with skepticism and defensiveness regarding the use of play. They inevitably progress to coming in, smiling, taking off their suit and tie, and asking, "What will we use to play today?" Other adults have commented, "for whatever reason, use of these activities helps me more than when we just talk."

In work I have done with couples, play therapy make it visually clearer to the partners what each individual wants in the relationship. It also helps clarify things for each individual about themselves while having their partner as a witness to their insight. Many couples who have come to treatment with me have had profound moments of understanding of what their partner has been trying to express for years, once they utilized play in expressing their thoughts and feelings. The use of play therapy and activities can be helpful to clients of any age who are either too heavily reliant on verbal communication and logic, and have difficulty accessing their emotions, as well as for those who have difficulty putting their thoughts, feelings, and/or experiences into verbal words.

Mary Anne Peabody, EdD, RPT-S

Bruner (1976) stated that play holds a critical developmental role for humans and I wholeheartedly agree. With a background in therapeutic recreation, I was introduced to play across the life span very early in my career as a way to promote healthy physical, intellectual, social, and emotional development. I am fascinated by social shifts in human play behavior as we move through different developmental ages and stage. Working now mostly with adults, I am intrigued that many adults need to give themselves permission to play (Walsh, 2019) and how adults often create excuses or alibis to justify playing socially (Deterding, 2018). As play therapists who play for our career, we may forget that some adults have difficulty playing.

My fascination with play across the life span was furthered fueled during my doctoral studies, when I completed a mini-field work experience with the Strong Children's Museum in Rochester, New York. Along with being a very unique children's museum, they are home to a vast library collection of play studies literature. Additionally, the museum publishes the American Journal of Play®, which is a scholarly peer-reviewed journal that synthesizes a variety of interdisciplinary perspectives to increase awareness and understanding of the role of play throughout human development. In my opinion all play therapists need to first understand play, just as all surgeons need to first understand general medicine. So, I strongly advocate for both play and play therapy understanding.

My clinical practice is now small and consists of volunteering with a small number of child clients. Even so, I continue to introduce play-based experiential learning with most parents during both the initial parent consultation meeting and if appropriate during family play therapy. The majority of my professional life is focused on teaching, research, and writing. My current research agenda explores the andragogical practices of play in higher education (James & Nerantzi, 2019). I study and practice a variety of playful andragogical practices in my teaching to serve as a model of how adult play is vital to development. In my teaching of play therapy to future play therapists, I believe students should experience the power inherent in play-based learning prior to asking children, parents or families to engage in play-based interventions, therefore I am very often engaged in play-based practices with those graduate students. Lastly, I also teach a freshman orientation course on play across the life span using some of the interpersonal neurobiology principles from Badenoch (2008) and Kestly (2014).

Dee Ray, PhD, RPT-S

Play is central component of being human and hence, an effective part of therapy across the life span. For my youngest clients who are below the age of 3, I primarily use child-parent relationship therapy (CPRT; Landreth & Bratton, 2019) in which I teach parents skills for play sessions with their children. CPRT is based on the premise that children's primary caretakers are the most effective change agents for their children, especially young children. When children reach 3 years old, I choose between child-centered play therapy and CPRT as principal interventions based on presenting issue and parent-child relationship dynamics. I typically facilitate traditional child-centered play therapy with 3- to 10-year-old children (Ray, 2011) due to the primacy of play as their language. As children reach preadolescence, I begin to experiment with the use of expressive arts structured activities as a modality that allows maturing children to integrate their new cognitive and verbal abilities with their most comfortable language of play.

Although we concentrate on play with children because play serves as their primary language, adolescents and adults may benefit from the use of play in overcoming their resistance to processing, accessing emotions and experiences that are difficult to identify, and integrating an active component to therapy. With adolescents and adults, I frequently use expressive arts structured activities as a regular part of therapy. I am especially partial to sand tray therapy (Homeyer & Sweeney, 2017) and will typically introduce sand tray to all adolescent and adult clients in order to explore their receptivity to and effectiveness with this medium. In using expressive arts structured activities, I attempt to match the client's style and comfort level with different mediums. For me, the use of play across the life span is the language mechanism to build the therapeutic relationship. More important than any play activity is my facilitation of a relationship that leads to healing and change. Play is the tool to build that relationship.

Jessica Stone, PhD, RPT-S

My practice includes approximately 40–50% children, 30–40% adolescents, 10% young adults, and 10% adults at any given time. Clearly there is an ebb and flow to the percentages, depending on the configuration of the people who come in. I find this balance to be a very good fit for me.

I have read articles, blogs, and posts about many people using play therapy with adults very successfully. This has not been my experience. Some adults over the years have been open to the idea of creating a traditional sand tray from time to time, but not many. For the most part, adults and adolescents have not wanted to engage with most play materials. Some adolescents appreciate board game play to deintensify the dyadic interaction; some will participate in drawing activities or some more structured craft creations; but others will not engage at all.

Some of the structured projects are fantastic if they will participate. A favorite of mine is to have the adolescent create a list of the things swarming around in their head. Often these will be texted over time and then the therapist can compile them, print them out, and together they concepts can be cut out. Separate pieces of paper can be used to organize these thoughts. For instance, a paper can be labeled as "school" and all the thoughts related to school can be taped/glued to the school paper. The concepts can be more global or specific depending on the needs of the client.

The therapeutic inclusion of technology has helped immensely with people who are averse to the more traditional forms of play. If a person does not want to draw in a traditional sense, perhaps a virtual reality session of Tilt Brust or SculptVR can provide another medium. If a person does not want to use the traditional sand tray, perhaps the Virtual Sandtray program would entice them. Additionally, if a person does not want to participate in relaxation strategies there are is an ever-growing list of relaxation/meditation virtual reality programs.

It is my experience that if you combine therapeutic benefit with a highly motivating activity, the result will be very beneficial for the treatment. The client will want to engage and will often provide a wealth of information within the activity, the play itself, the narration during, and/or the discussion afterward. Interventions which are vetted in advance, explored and determined to have therapeutic value, and available for all clients in a prescriptive manner will improve the quality and effectiveness of the therapeutic interactions for all ages.

Daniel Sweeney, PhD, RPT-S

The age range for play therapy spans from infancy through geriatrics. Since play therapy fundamentally involves the use of play as a means of therapeutic communication and connection, it is not limited for use with children. There is play therapy literature spanning from infancy (Courtney, 2020), adolescents (Gallo-Lopez & Schaefer, 2005), adults (Schaefer, 2003), and even geriatric clients (Mackenzie, James, Morse, Mukaetova-Ladinska, & Reichelt, 2006).

I primarily use CCPT with young children. The primary play therapy intervention that I use with preadolescents, adolescents, and adults is sand tray therapy (Homeyer & Sweeney, 2017). I have found this to be very effective clinically. Across ages, I also use other expressive arts interventions (e.g., clay, paints, mandalas, drawings, storytelling, puppets, and drama).

I have worked with a wide age range of clients, from toddlers to clients in their 70s. I do not have much experience with the geriatric population. I have worked with a wide range of psychiatric diagnoses, from the "classic" childhood diagnoses (attention deficit hyperactivity disorder (ADHD), reactive attachment disorder (RAD), oppositional defiant disorder (ODD), conduct disorder (CD), disruptive mood dysregulation disorder (DMDD)) to severe anxiety, depression, autism, personality disorders, and so on. Play therapy has often been the primary intervention or an auxiliary intervention. It is an effective and needed intervention across the life span.

References

Badenoch, B. (2008). *Being a brain-wise therapist: A practical guide to interpersonal neurobiology.* Norton.

Bruner, J. S. (1976). Nature and uses of immaturity. In J. S. Bruner, A. Jolly, & K. Sylva (Eds.), *Play: Its role in development and evolution* (pp. 28–64). Basic Books.

Caldwell, C. (2003). Adult group play therapy. In C. E. Schaefer (Ed.), *Play therapy with adults.* John Wiley & Sons, Inc.

Courtney, J. (Ed.). (2020). *Infant play therapy: Foundations, models, programs, and practice.* Routledge.

Deterding, S. (2018). Alibis for adult play: A Goffmanian account of escaping embarrassment in adult play. *Games and Culture, 13*(3), 260–279.

Erikson, E. H. (1993, 1950). *Childhood and society.* W.W. Norton & Company. (p.242).

Fuss, A. (2010). *Client-centered play therapy with an elderly assisted living facility resident.* http://trace.tennessee.edu/cgi/viewcontent.cgi?article=1622&context=utk_graddiss

Gallo-Lopez, L., & Schaefer, C. (Eds.). (2005). *Play therapy with adolescents.* Rowman & Littlefield Publishers.

Garrett, M. (2014). Beyond play therapy: Using the sandtray as an expressive arts intervention in counseling adult clients. *Asia Pacific Journal of Counselling and Psychotherapy, 5*(1), 99–105.

Gass, M. A., Gillis, H. L., & Russell, K. C. (2012). *Adventure therapy: Theory, research, and practice.* Routledge.

Green, E. J. (2010, June). Jungian play therapy with adolescents. *Play Therapy, 5*(2), 20–23.

Green, E. J., Drewes, A. A., & Kominski, J. M. (2013). Use of mandalas in Jungian play therapy with adolescents diagnosed with ADHD. *International Journal of Play Therapy, 22*(3), 159–172.

Green, E. J., Baggerly, J., & Myrick, A. (2018). *Play therapy with preteens.* Rowman & Littlefield.

Homeyer, L., & Sweeney, D. (2017). Sandtray therapy: A practical manual (3rd ed.). Routledge.

Kaduson, H. G. (2016). Play therapy across the life span: Infants, children, adolescents and adults. In K. J. O'Connor, C. E. Schaefer, & L. D. Braverman (Eds.). *Handbook of play therapy* (2nd ed., pp. 327–342). Wiley.

Kestly, T. A. (2014). *The interpersonal neurobiology of play.* W.W. Norton & Company.

James, A., & Nerantzi, C. (2019). *The power of play in higher education: Creativity in tertiary learning.* Palgrave McMillian.

Landreth, G., & Bratton, S. (2019). *Child-parent relationship therapy: An evidence-based 10 session filial model* (2nd ed.). Routledge.

Lindaman, S. (1994). Geriatric theraplay. In C. E. Kevin & J. O'Connor (Eds.), *Handbook of play therapy* (Vol. II, pp. 207–228). John Wiley & Sons, Inc.

Mackenzie, L., James, I., Morse, R., Mukaetova-Ladinska, E., & Reichelt, F. (2006). A pilot study on the use of dolls for people with dementia. *Age and Ageing, 35*(4), 441–444.

Olson-Morrison, D. (2017). Integrative play therapy with adults with complex trauma: A developmentally-informed approach. *International Journal of Play Therapy, 26*(3), 177–183.

Piaget, J. (1936). *Origins of Intelligence in the Child.* Routledge & Kegan Paul.

Ray, D. (2011). *Advanced play therapy: Essential conditions, knowledge, and skills for child practice.* Routledge.

Schaefer, C. E. (2003). *Play therapy with adults.* Wiley.

Schaefer, C. E., & Gallo-Lopez, L. (Eds.). (2010). *Play therapy with adolescents.* Jason Aronson.

Schaefer, C. E., Kelly-Zion, P., McCormick, J., & Ohnogi, A. (Eds.). (2008). *Play therapy with very young children.* Rowman & Littlefield.

Walsh, A. (2019). Giving permission for adults to play. *The Journal of Play in Adulthood, 1*(1), 1–14.

Ward-Wimmer, D. (2003). The healing potential of adults at play. In C. E. Schaefer & C. Westland (Eds.), *Playing, living, learning: A worldwide perspective on children's opportunities to play.* Venture Publishing.

Conclusion

Clair Mellenthin and Jessica Stone

In play therapy supervision and training, I often tell individuals, "there is no wrong way to do play therapy, unless you are causing harm", meaning as long as you are grounded in theory and practicing from an ethical standpoint, it is so important and critical to the longevity of your clinical career to find your own voice and be your authentic self in the process. As the old saying goes, you truly are the most important toy in the playroom, regardless of what theoretical orientation speaks to you and makes the most sense in your work with children and families. Showing up as your authentic self is what will make the difference in your caseload and with the children whose paths you are blessed to cross.

Throughout the pages of this book, our hope is that you have found that there are several ways of thinking about, practicing, and implementing play therapy. There can be a sense of confusion at times in the field of play therapy as there are many different theories and perspectives on how to do this great work. As you have read through these chapters, you will have heard competing voices as well as complementary factors that arise even when theoretical perspectives differ. Our shared hope and vision for this book is to provide a bridge of understanding, that the sharing our differences can be a strength to our field and not a division. Play *is* universal, as is our shared goals of making a difference in the lives of the children and families we work with.

– Clair Mellenthin

Play Therapy Theories and Perspectives provides responses from ten credentialed play therapists which highlight both the diversity and similarities in each practitioner's approach. The play therapy umbrella is broad and allows for the customization of conceptualization and implementation. Grounded in experience, the play therapists highlighted within these pages answer questions in each of the text's main categories: perspectives, process, and practice.

Early and seasoned therapists alike will benefit from hearing the perspectives of each clinician, whether it be to broaden one's views or support and/ or complement existing positions. The power of learning about how others conceptualize cases, choose and apply theory, and address challenges will inform the reader's practice and professional growth. As Robert has stated in the introduction, "Although unity in play therapy is evident, there still exists diversity in approach and thought. Diversity and differences do not have to be considered problematic. In fact, they are assets that enrich the professional experience. Diversity and differing perspectives contribute to the strengths in creating the best possible format in which to provide therapy", the importance of both unity and diversity cannot be underemphasized.

We truly appreciate the time and attention you have afforded each of the pages within this book. Perhaps you have been inspired to answer the questions for yourself. Hopefully the readings have prompted you to identify which areas under the play therapy umbrella are your strengths and which areas might need more exploration. A commitment to respecting differences, understanding and appreciating unity and diversity, valuing and expanding perspectives, and a celebration of differences will solidify all of us as play therapists who are dedicated to provide excellent treatment for our clients. Whatever your sentiment(s), may your journey within play therapy be inspirational, exciting, and stimulating!

– Jessica Stone

Index

Note: **Bold** page numbers refer to tables and *italic* page numbers refer to figures.